SO YOU'VE REGISTERED, WHAT NOW?

A NEW NURSE'S GUIDE

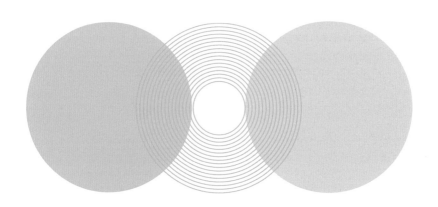

SO YOU'VE REGISTERED, WHAT NOW?

A NEW NURSE'S GUIDE

JOLEEN McKEE, RN (Adult), BSc (Hons)
Ulster University
Nursing Development Lead
Belfast Health and Social Care Trust
RCN Learning Representative

ELSEVIER

ELSEVIER

SO YOU'VE REGISTERED, WHAT NOW?:
A NEW NURSE'S GUIDE

ISBN: 978-0-3239-3392-6

Content Strategist: Robert Edwards
Content Development Specialist: Denise Roslonski
Content Development Director: Laurie Gower
Publishing Services Manager: Shereen Jameel
Project Manager: Haritha Dharmarajan
Designer: Patrick Ferguson

Working together
to grow libraries in
developing countries

www.elsevier.com • www.bookaid.org

Printed in Poland

Last digit is the print number: 9   8   7   6   5   4   3   2   1

CONTENTS

Making the transition to your role as a registered nurse can be an exciting but scary prospect. The sense of anticipation is great; this is what you worked for. Now is the time to put those hard-won skills and capabilities, knowledge and expertise to the test. As a young staff nurse, I recall the sense of trepidation even though I knew I was fortunate to be in an environment which was vibrant, buzzy and had the benefit of superb clinical leadership. Even with those assets it's still daunting, which is why it is important to reach out for that helping hand wherever you can find it. That is what I think Joleen has provided in this book; a companion, a fellow travelogue to tune into as you navigate your way in this new world. It does this by drawing on the experience of someone who has recently been there herself; understands the ups and downs. The tone is peer to peer, like 'talking to a friend'. Let's face it, we need friends to support us in everything we do. There are also a lot of practical tips to help guide you as a newly registered nurse through the channels of beginning a clinical career. As I look back on my career, I can see how the start we have at the beginning can be crucial to what comes next. This book helps you realise you are not alone; many of your concerns are shared by others. That can be a comfort and consolation. Most important of all, if you need help or support ask for it and ask quickly – it will save you needless angst and anxiety. Don't struggle alone. These are great rules to live by when starting out and will stand you in good stead as you move through your career and support others. So, I commend this guide to you and wish you every success in what I hope is a dazzling career to come.

Prof. Dame Anne Marie Rafferty
Past President of the RCN
Professor of Health & Nursing Policy
King's College London

It seems like yesterday.

The day I stood for the first time in front of a medicine trolley in a bay full of sleepy patients at 07:30 in the morning wearing my fresh, crisp, new blue uniform with the keys in my hand, a hand-over in my pocket and a lump in my throat. My first day as a newly registered nurse is a day I will never forget, not because I did anything extraordinary like saving a life with moments to spare or performing an emergency Heimlich, but because it was the first time a patient called me 'nurse' and I realised it was real.

All those years of hard work, studying and anticipation faded away in an instant. I was no longer the trainee, the intern, the student; now I had my PIN and 'Registered Nurse' written across my chest. I felt indestructible, yet fragile. I remember that day so clearly, the first time I checked a drug with another nurse, the first time a doctor came to me planning a patient's discharge, the first time a family member thanked me for caring for their loved one and the first time I gave hand-over, alone. Yes, I had completed all of these tasks many times as a student, but this was the first time I didn't have a mentor to guide me every step of the way. I did it on my own and I was so proud. I still am.

As the days, months and years have passed, I still think back to my first day. Those feelings of true excitement, passion and determination to be the best nurse I can be as well as the tremendous worry and anxiety that I felt. Yes, I had a great preceptor and a fabulous team of nurses where I worked, but in reality it took being on my own to make me realise that I could do it. I could be a nurse, and so can you.

Today, nursing is faced with so many challenges, too many to mention here, but what will never change is how much a smile can change a patient's day, how much a listening ear can reassure someone during their darkest times, and how much this profession really and truly gives you much more than you can ever imagine.

You've made the right choice. Being a nurse is pretty incredible.

On that first day all those years ago, I never imagined how my career would change so much. I didn't think I would be sitting here writing a preface for a book to help guide the next generation of nurses. It just goes to show how varied and surprising this profession really is.

In this book, we will go on a journey together. We will discuss how to get your first job, how to become a reflective practitioner, how to be a mentor, and how to survive and thrive in your new career. The journey you are about to embark upon as a newly registered nurse may feel daunting, but we will get through this… together.

This book is not meant to be a definitive guide to nursing. If you are reading this, then chances are you will be studying or have studied the theory and practice of the profession. Rather, it is a handbook, an opening of the door into your new world of what it means to be a real nurse today.

So let's begin.

Joleen McKee (2023)

ACKNOWLEDGEMENTS

To Chris, my wonderful partner in crime. Thank you for being my biggest supporter and always believing in me even when I had lost faith in myself. You truly are my soulmate, and I pinch myself every day that I have you in my life.

To my wonderful family, thank you for always being there and supporting me in everything I do.

To my mother Ann, you may not be a nurse by profession, but you have taught me so much about nursing, more than you will ever realize. You instilled in me the values of care and compassion from a young age and have helped shape me into the person I am today. Thank you for being you.

To my father Joe, thank you for showing me that the only way to deal with challenges is to face them head on. I am so proud of you each and every day.

To my sister Anna, you have always been there for me, and I know you always will be, and for that I am forever thankful.

To my brother Joseph, I am so proud of the man and the father you have become.

To my beautiful niece Aoife, my aunt Tracie and my brother-in-law Chris, and my other close friends and relatives, thank you for your support and guidance throughout my life so far.

To my precious dog Minnie, who has always brightened my day, no matter how hard it has been.

To Chris
Without you, none of this would have been possible. Thank you
for making my dreams come true.

SO YOU'VE REGISTERED, WHAT NOW?

A NEW NURSE'S GUIDE

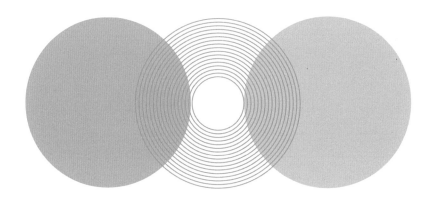

CHAPTER 1

And So the Journey Begins

In life, every great journey has to start somewhere. In this case it was your eureka moment, that realisation that you had a calling to become a nurse and to dedicate your life to helping others. For some, it happens at a young age. For others, life experience or the kindness that they were shown by another nurse helped ignite that fire inside them to follow the same path.

Let's think back to your first day as a student nurse. Do you remember the nervous excitement you felt? That electric energy you had as you put on your fresh, crisp new uniform, and your thoughts about what the future would hold? Now, here we are, a little older and a lot wiser, and once again we think about what lies ahead as we prepare to don a new uniform. Perhaps it's a tunic; maybe it's army fatigues or even a simple shirt. Whatever the outfit, the key difference this time is your name badge and the words 'registered nurse' written across your chest.

It may seem as though you went from being the student with a mentor to rely on to the nurse in charge of actual patients on your own in no time. Exciting, isn't it? Or is terrifying a more accurate representation of how you are currently feeling? In reality you've done it, you've achieved your end goal, you've worked so hard and sacrificed so much to get here. Don't let the fears and doubts get in the way of what can be an amazing journey.

At this point you've already opened the gate and are on your way. The preparation and skills gained from your nurse training should provide the foundation blocks to build upon.

Starting a new job can be frustrating for anyone, whatever the profession. However, fear not, you will be okay. Unlike people entering most other jobs, you have a head start on being able to adapt to new areas, different teams and fresh challenges. You've done this all before; think back to the many times you were the new person on placement and all of the feelings of excitement yet that nervous energy you felt. Do those memories feel similar to how you are feeling now? From the moment you entered the lecture hall or stepped foot into a daunting placement, you were preparing for where you are right now. Let's take a look at some of your worries one by one.

I was so confident when I was a student, but now that I am actually qualified and out working on my own, I feel like a deer caught in the headlights.

Stop right here. Take a deep breath. Feeling like this is normal. You will feel overwhelmed, you will feel like you can't do it, but all those years of hard slog in your nursing degree prove to you that you can and that you will. There are many things you don't know and so much more that you do. This stage of your career is about learning, about adapting and about finding out what type of nurse you want to be. Don't expect too much from yourself. Yes, some colleagues will outrank your experience. Even some of your fellow newly registered class may give an air of confidence that you have yet to master, but Rome was not built in a day, and your nursing journey will not be defined by those early days. Allow yourself to grow into it. No one is expecting you to show up on your first day and run the show.

What your colleagues will expect

- You will know and follow your department's policies and procedures
- You are punctual and ready for your shift
- You are polite and professional and understand how you should communicate with colleagues and patients
- You understand how to be a team player

In terms of your skill set, your colleagues will expect

- You understand and can carry out the basic fundamentals of nursing
- You can recognise and respond to a deteriorating patient
- You are competent in medication management
- You will know when to ask questions and when to request help

These lists should not come as a surprise. Some of them translate to every area of work; competence, punctuality, being respectful, appreciating that you will not nor be expected to know it all. Are they expectations which differ from your life, perhaps mere months ago, as a final-year studying nursing?

There is one difference, of course: the level of responsibility which now rests on your shoulders. But, to repeat it again, you've got this. Although the skills and expectation levels will be similar from your placement days, now you are more accountable and need to 'step up' to be the nurse you wanted to be when you set off on your journey. The stabilisers are off; now your ride can begin.

I don't feel ready, what happens if something goes badly wrong? Will the Nursing and Midwifery Council (NMC) get involved?

There comes a point in every nursing career when you have to trust your training and believe in your instincts. And there is no better time for this than when you are first setting out. As a newly registered nurse, you should be up to speed on the latest standards and the most up-to-date methods. If you are not, you need to address this, or ask for help. Sometimes it can be the more experienced nursing staff who could be liable to make mistakes, mostly through complacency about updating their skills or pridefully thinking they are immune to making errors.

Always remember that to err is human, but if you are unsure, always, always, ask for help. You will likely be judged for making a mistake, but good colleagues should be understanding if you ask for help before this happens.

Avoid

1. **Being the big shot:** Don't act like you know more than what you do. Be honest and proud of your skill set; people will respect that more than pretending you know more than you do and making mistakes just to try and 'show off'. No one appreciates arrogance in the workplace.
2. **Having scatter brain:** Make sure to be organised and have a rough plan for your day. Don't try to have a photographic memory; you will forget things that may be super important. Make plans, create notes and tick off your to-dos as you go so you know what to prioritise.
3. **Crashing and burning:** Nurse burnout is a real thing and a pretty big deal. We will touch on burnout later in the book, but just remember to take time for yourself and always tell someone that you're struggling with your workload or the pressures you are facing. There is always help out there; you just have to ask for it.

Coming up, we will discuss ways in which you can deal with the risk of burnout and the stresses which come from your daily life as a nurse. For now, let's park that. Instead, focus on these simple rules for what you should do if you make a mistake. The same as in normal life, small mistakes can eat away at your confidence. Big mistakes can feel like you would rather a hole in the ground opened up for you to step into. Really though, it doesn't have to be the end of the world, even if, in the moment, it can feel that way.

Try these

The patient is number one: Ultimately, you care for them, they are the priority and above all else, whether a mistake has been committed or not, their health and well-being are in your hands. You owe it to them and the profession to make sure they trust that their care is top quality. You will be surrounded in your workplace by senior colleagues, many of whom will have seen more testing scenarios than you will encounter in your early years as a nurse. Let them guide you and be a calming influence so you can refocus and put the patient's needs first. Mistakes can be analysed later, but in the moment, always make sure they are addressed with the patient at the centre.

Hold your hands up: Honesty really is the best policy. If you make a mistake, own up straight away. Be open and clear about how the mistake was made, and communicate everything so that if a patient's health is potentially at risk, then your colleagues have all the information they need to help you find a solution.

Don't dwell on it, learn from it: In the moment, mistakes can feel soul-destroying and harm your confidence. However, few people reach the top or become the best without making mistakes and then finding ways to improve by learning from them. Some of the great advancements in nursing will have come from trial and error or through lessons learned. None of us are perfect, and there is a reason why reflection forms not only a key part of this book but an essential part of daily nursing; it is because it is vital to your understanding of what the job demands and how we can always improve. So don't let a mistake eat you up. Devour it, and let it motivate you to be the best nurse you can be.

As far as the NMC getting involved, it really all depends on the mistake. For most cases, small lapses in judgement or things that can be easily resolved, it is unlikely that they will ever cross the NMC's desk. For the bigger things, they may need to be notified. At the end of the day, the NMC is there to help protect the public and support nurses; it is not the 'Big Bad Wolf' you picture in your head. If you stick to your training, provide care that is backed by evidence and always ask for help when you need it, then you should have nothing to worry about. It will often be more experienced nurses who are more likely to be called in front of the NMC. This may be as a result of complacency and carelessness in keeping skills and knowledge fresh. This could happen to you, someday.

If you take one thing away from this chapter, or indeed the whole book, it is about focus and fighting against complacency. Just because you have graduated and registered does not mean you stop being a student of nursing. It is a role that for every generation of nurses has demanded an evolution to handle developing medicines, techniques, patient behaviour and the stresses and strains with staffing pressures and morale. The author of this book did not expect a global pandemic to strike within a few years of collecting her pin, and whatever environment you enter when reading this book, be prepared that you could face challenges we have yet to even contemplate.

But… remember this: we nurses are in this together. So, ask for help, keep yourself right by the guidelines, retain that inquisitive student mentality, and there will, hopefully, never be a need for the NMC to blow your house down.

What if they don't accept me as a nurse?

Let's think about that statement for a second. What if your new colleagues don't accept you as a nurse; is this really about them or you? Are you worrying deep down that you aren't ready to be a nurse? It's obvious from your experience as a student that it isn't going to be easy; in fact, it can be really difficult at times and you will feel like you want to give up. Remember how many times you felt this way during your training? Did you give up? No, you continued on through all of the stress, the long days and sleepless nights shifts. Why? Because you became a nurse the day you decided that this was your career, that nursing was your calling.

To help you through this feeling, here are a few suggestions

Everyone has a role to play; respect everyone regardless of their position: It is pretty cool that you have gone from the student who everyone tells what to do to the nurse in charge of actual staff members. Despite that, you must always remember where you started. You are no better than any other member of the team because you are a nurse. Be willing to learn from everyone, including those you outrank.

Delegate appropriately: Don't expect others to do your work for you; work as a team and help your colleagues out when you can.

Always ask for help: Don't be worried about what others think; they were you once and probably asked the same questions you're thinking of. Those who don't ask questions or for help are doomed to never learn from, and are likely to repeat, their mistakes.

It may seem odd that this book starts off by highlighting the pitfalls and risks of mistake. It is merely to set out that you should not fear failure as you begin your nursing journey. Accept that sometimes mistakes will happen, but be alert to them. Do not let the fear of error make you shy away from doing your utmost for your patient. It may take you longer than others, but eventually every nurse will find their voice and their confidence. You did not make the decision to study and register lightly; this is not like any other job. So do not be frightened; you have a long road ahead and it will be as rewarding as it is challenging.

Everyone asks the same questions. Whether it's like you, before starting your first job, or after 20 years' experience, the first things we all think about are:

- Will my mistakes haunt me?
- Am I good enough?
- Will my colleagues respect me?

Nursing is a learning process. Be confident, but don't expect to be an expert from day one. Look around at your experienced colleagues. They were you once, and some day you will be them, watching as the newly registered nurses step onto the ward and helping them with tasks you once asked for support with.

The Nursing Workforce Community

There are so many roles in the nursing workforce community, all equally important. You may have started off working as a healthcare assistant, then you became 'the student' and now here you are the newly registered nurse and soon you'll be the senior nurse, possibly a charge nurse or a ward manager. One day we may even call you the director of nursing or the chief nursing officer. Wow! So much scope, so much learning, and what an adventure it's going to be.

One thing to remember during this exciting journey is how you feel right now. That fearful excitement of being new, fresh and ready to take on the world. To do the right thing for your patients and the passion you have to be the best nurse you can. To make a difference no matter how small.

Working as a nurse today can make it extremely hard to keep these feelings and experiences at the forefront of our minds. You, a newly registered nurse, already have fears, doubts and worries about being good enough or ready to take on your new role. But, with the added pressures the healthcare systems currently face, including lack of resources, funds, an ageing population, evolving healthcare needs and the continuous problem of safe staffing levels, not to mention a global pandemic thrown in for good measure, it's hard to remember why you started.

Each member of the team, from the student setting out on the journey to the consultant, administration staff, domestics and more, has a vital role to play. One cannot care for the patient in isolation. To use a sport analogy, we're specialists in our own positions, and while you cannot win a match by playing only defence or attack, we must pull together and respect what each of us brings if we are to stand a chance of success.

Workplace cliques and talking about a colleague behind their back bring no benefits, only a disjointed environment lacking in trust…and we all know in nursing you really do need to trust your colleagues during those difficult moments.

Other members of the multidisciplinary team play a tremendous role in teaching others about their area of expertise. For example, you have a patient with a tracheostomy. You've completed your relevant training and feel like you're doing well, but suctioning secretions from a tracheotomy scares you a little. That's okay; that's a normal way to feel at first. Suctioning for the first time can feel a little overwhelming, especially when you're new to this particular skill; it is the patient's airway after all, and you're responsible for keeping it clear. So to help you build confidence in this area, why not ask the physiotherapist to show you how they suction? Ask for hints and tips. Ask the physiotherapist to observe your technique, and before you know it you'll be teaching someone else your newfound skills.

As a nurse, you are part of the nursing team but also part of the wider setup which contributes to a patient's care. It is no better nor worse a role than the others, but an equally vital cog in the wheel.

The same goes for your health care assistant, your domestic staff, your catering assistants—could you really do your job without them? So always remember, we are all working together as part of one team with the goal of creating good patient experiences and helping each other out along the way. No one is more superior than someone else because of a job title; everyone deserves respect.

You might be worried, but you do have the ability to take on this new role. If you were a competent and safe final-year student (and let's face it, if you've got this far, you must have been), then you are a competent and safe newly registered nurse. Don't let your doubts and fears distract you from the joy and personal growth that awaits you in your new career.

So let's dive in….

CHAPTER 2

So You've Registered, What Now?

A nursing qualification can be a passport to the world and a ticket to open many doors at home. It is a vocation which is so revered and necessary that the opportunities for personal growth, career development and great experiences are seemingly endless. One guarantee is that no two days will be the same.

Take a second and think: Was there a moment you realised nursing was for you? Was it always in the cards, or have you changed your mind more times than you care to count?

Ask a fellow nurse, why they made the same decision and listen carefully to the reasons they give; you might be surprised at what motivates your colleagues. Some may say with emotion that they 'wanted to help people'. Others may be more practical and scientific with their answers and explain their fascination with the human body and how illness, disease, the environment or the world around us affects everyday existence. Perhaps your colleague entered nursing because their father was a nurse. Maybe it was because of the care their mother received that prompted them to see their future differently. On a lighter note, I guess we all know that few will enter nursing for the money.

As nurses, we have so much opportunity to work in multiple different areas throughout our careers, but getting started can feel as though you've tried to ride a bike for the first time with the stabilisers off. Let this chapter metaphorically act as those stabilisers. Allow it to help guide you through the minefield of job opportunities and the decisions you need to make about where to work. So, let's take an adventure together and explore the various opportunities this wonderful profession has to offer you.

Hospital Nursing

There is a good chance that you have had first-hand experience of nursing in a hospital, especially from undertaking placements during your degree. It goes without saying that from the point of entry, a patient can encounter a nurse from the emergency department (ED) door to the surgical theatres and the recovery wards. At every stage of their journey, nurses are at the core of hospital care.

When thinking about work in this area, consider your emotions from placements. Did it feel like home? Was the work challenging or too intense? In this setting, you will witness and treat some incredibly sick patients, including those who, through no fault of our own, may not make it back out of hospital. You will encounter families traumatised or saddened, or also extremely grateful for the care you provide. Others may be tense and seek confrontation with the nursing staff.

Hospital life truly defines the saying that no two days are the same. But it can also mean working with tight-knit staffing groups who will trust each other with life-and-death moments, often under circumstances where staffing is short. It can be both inspirational and frustrating. There will be long hours and times when, like many other nursing jobs, it can be hard to switch off once you leave the wards. That image of a patient you know has hours left to live. Or the heart warmth that comes from the hug offered from an appreciative relative. There are many things that will stick in your mind.

The areas you can work in at a hospital are varied: for example, medical wards and admissions, surgical wards, theatres, intensive care units (ICU), EDs, outpatient departments, and specialist care centres, such as cancer care. The list goes on and on.

Rotation Programmes

Let's take a look at a possibility for those who simply can't choose where they want to begin their careers. Have you ever considered or heard of a rotation programme?

Most trusts these days offer rotation programmes that allow nurses to explore different areas usually within the same organisation for six months up to two years so they can gain skills and build confidence in multiple specialities. These rotation programmes offer exposure to a wide range of clinical skills. They can help individuals to clarify career paths, improve their resilience and build up their confidence and leadership capabilities.

Although most rotations typically focus on clinical placements, some also offer non-clinical opportunities to include research and development.

Think of the rotation programme like a box of chocolates that is being shared among your family. You look down at the little menu card to find the one you want, but in reality there are several you'd love to sample. In a rotation programme, you have the option to indulge by selecting a few different areas that interest you and see if one of them is somewhere you could see yourself working longer-term.

Let's take a look at Linda's story.

Linda chose to become a nurse because of the care she witnessed being given to a family member while they were in the ICU. Therefore, it was a clear first option when Linda chose to opt for a rotation programme when she registered. However, after a placement during her degree in the ED, Linda realised she was an adrenaline junkie and loved the fast pace and the varied nature of the patients she saw coming through the doors every shift. ED soon became her second choice on her rotation. Linda also chose general surgery, not because she loved surgical wounds (in fact, Linda wasn't a fan of this type of nursing and didn't feel a ward-based job was for her), but because she had heard this is a great area for skill development. She felt this experience would be beneficial for her possible new role in ICU or ED.

From the moment I decided I wanted to become a nurse, it was only ICU or ED I could ever see myself working in. I know it's weird to say, but I really thrive looking after extremely sick patients and I felt I could only get that adrenaline fix working in one of these high-intensity areas. As my rotation went on, I felt so burnt out, and things just didn't feel right for some reason. I had this overwhelming feeling that I wasn't making the right decision by basing my choices on what I thought I wanted. It got to my last placement on the rotation which was general surgery, and I was honestly dreading it. I had only chosen it to fill a gap. I just didn't think I was cut out for the routine of ward-based nursing. I was so wrong. General surgery has taught me that you really don't know what you want until you try it out, and now I couldn't be happier.

(LINDA ANDREWS, GENERAL SURGERY NURSE)

Linda's story shows us that sometimes we may think that we really want to work in a particular area, but actually working there isn't what we had expected after all.

Georgina, who works in London, is another nurse who wasn't sure which area she wanted to work in when she registered, so she also opted for a rotation programme.

She said completing the rotation programme gave her *'so many unique learning and growth opportunities'.*

'Although I work in a highly specialist hospital, each workplace was memorable for its own reasons. I had different role models to learn from and saw a variety of patients with specific care needs. Similar to my time as a nursing student, I became an expert at being the new nurse'. Georgina says working in different teams and routines helped her to become more aware of her practice and *'the rationale behind what we do and why we do them'.*

The experience she gained was valuable, although it does mean some adjustment is needed to adapt to new teams. She cited an example that flummoxed her new colleagues in a respiratory ward when she rotated from cardiology. In cardiology, electrocardiograms (ECGs) were completed by the night team so they were ready for the day shift staff.

So doing this became routine while on nightshift. When I was on the respiratory ward, I remember wheeling the ECG machine to a patient just as I was coming to the end of my shift. This patient was having daily ECGs, but as I went to carry this out, my colleagues actually thought there was an emergency and came to help.

Georgina says she remembers them being 'mortified' that she would consider waking up a patient for an ECG that could be performed by the day team.

Georgina, who now works as a paediatric nurse in a high-dependency department in London, says her experience as a newly registered nurse and the skills and knowledge she gained during her rotation programme helped her to transition back into the role of an adult nurse when she was called upon for redeployment during the COVID-19 pandemic.

I am now a paediatric nurse, so things are very different, from drug doses to how we carry out and analyse simple examinations like blood pressure. Without my rotation experience I would not have felt confident to nurse adults again. I was able to draw upon what I had learnt during this time to help me transition into this new role. Nursing COVID-19 patients was so diverse, we all needed to use various skills, so having had experience in multiple different areas was great, I felt I had an advantage to some of my other colleagues who had only ever worked in one particular area before.

(GEORGINA LEDWITH, PAEDIATRIC NURSE-COMPLETED A ROTATION IN CARDIOLOGY, RESPIRATORY, AND MEDICAL ADMISSIONS AS AN ADULT NURSE)

As the case studies above highlight, there are some great benefits to beginning your career in a rotation programme. It offers the experience of sampling different areas, enhancing both your skills and knowledge. However, as Georgina's example shows, there can be challenges in adjusting from one area to the next.

For many people hospital nursing can be a fascinating start to their nursing journey, while for others it may not be their cup of tea. So, for those of you who could never picture starting your career in a hospital setting, let's explore what options are out there.

Primary Care

Many people believe nursing is synonymous with the hospital and ward environments, but of course, there is no such thing as a natural habitat for our line of work. Some nurses will work in primary care, which can involve general practice (GP), schools or at a variety of health clinics, such as ophthalmology. Primary care is another line of defence along the health care front line. Of course, we should expect to find nurses there.

Jayne is a registered nurse working in her local ophthalmology clinic that treats patients with all sorts of eye problems.

At our clinic, we treat patients with various eye conditions from macular degeneration to cataracts and sight difficulties as a result of stroke or neurological conditions. When I was training as a nurse, I never realised the scope of practice we really have. Working in 'eyes' wasn't an area I had ever considered, mostly because it wasn't something I was familiar with, but when I started working here, I realised just how much this area relates to so many other conditions. At our clinic we offer a range of treatments, and our nurse practitioners even offer eye injections to help maintain a patient's sight. We take medical histories just as you would on a ward admission and even insert cannulas and obtain blood for specific tests. Nursing really is so versatile and there are so many options out there, you just have to think outside the box sometimes.

(JAYNE MCKEOWN, STAFF NURSE OPHTHALMOLOGY)

When we think primary care, what we really mean is public health or community nursing. It brings in a wide range of services that are delivered outside of an acute care setting. Community nursing, such as district nursing, is one of the biggest sectors within primary care.

These nurses provide an invaluable service to patients at their homes who require nursing assistance: anything from wound and diabetes management to catheter insertions and blood sampling. Community nurses also assist in providing patients with complex care in areas such as palliative care. Florence is a newly registered community nurse; this is her story.

Community Nursing

It's kinda like getting hit by a train.

Florence, a community staff nurse in Devon, has been qualified for several months but still remembers the dread and fear of her first shift.

How the hell am I going to do this? How am I going to remember stuff? Even simple things like taking the right dressings to people's houses I was stressing about, she reflects.

In recent years, there has been a change whereby those who are newly qualified can enter community nursing as a first job, rather than needing experience elsewhere.

There can be a *'stigma'*, Florence suggests, around choosing the community first, rather than, for instance, a hospital setting.

A lot of people will be like, 'don't do it, you're going to de-skill', or once you go to community you won't get offered a job anywhere else, she says.
But I am so so glad I did it, I'm really enjoying it. I have 100% learned so much in the community.

There can be some 'bias', she adds, with each nurse believing their area of work is best.

However, the autonomy and variety of experiences in community nursing, Florence explains, can be *'quite daunting'*, but equally rewarding.

You just have to get on with it and you learn on the job.
There's always someone at the end of the phone, which I think is an important thing.

Florence says she sometimes rings her coordinator eight to 10 times a day and trusts there is support available if she needs it.

It is really important to be honest. If you get a visit on your list or something you're not confident in, always ask for help. I usually request another nurse to join me on that visit until I have mastered that particular skill.

Apart from learning how to manage your time well, one piece of advice I would urge all prospective community nurses to heed is, do not self-neglect'.

In her early weeks, Florence says she stopped meal-prepping and got into a rut with eating and drinking during her shifts. She also stopped seeing friends due to her dedication to the job.

During the COVID-19 pandemic, she says nurses in her area were offered the opportunity to undertake remote working that has helped her to go home every lunchtime for breaks.

Given the distance a community nurse can travel from appointment to appointment, Florence says to look after yourself first in such a role, even down to planning for toilet breaks.

Another part of the job, and something which all nurses can associate with, is the belief that upon qualifying, all nursing knowledge has gone out of the window and you do not feel confident to enter the world of work.

However, Florence says she surprised herself with how much information was underpinning her work, with nursing instincts rising to the fore when they were most needed. In Florence's case, knowing the right thing to say when having challenging conversations with palliative patients.

A lot of students will message me and say 'oh, I know nothing, university hasn't prepared me at all', but actually once they've started, deep down you have a lot more knowledge than you think you do.

As for job advice, Florence suggests there are many opportunities within community nursing, and employers are looking for candidates who 'can show that you are going to be a good autonomous practitioner and you're going to communicate well with your team'.

To find out more about Florence's experience as a community nurse, visit her Instagram account where she chronicles the daily emotions and joys of this type of nursing: @nursingwithflo.

Primary care shows how varied a career nursing can be and the range of ways we can treat patients, from the hospital to the home. Whether it is an option immediately after qualification or an area you wish to challenge yourself in down the line, there is no doubt how important a service this type of nursing is to the patient, so these are jobs worthy of your consideration.

Here is a list of primary care jobs you could research:

- GP practice nurse
- School nurse
- Prison nurse/Police custody nurse
- District/community nurse
- Rapid response nurse
- Home intravenous (IV) therapy nurse
- Heart failure nurse
- Diabetes nurse

- Wound care nurse
- Continence nurse
- Health visitor
- Sexual health and reproductive nurse
- Asthma nurse
- Outreach children's nurse
- Learning disability day centre nurse
- Community mental health nurse

The list goes on, and although some of these jobs may require additional training or some further experience, they are still options open to you during your career so take a look, you might find something you never would have considered before.

Care Homes

This is a unique setting for nursing care and has some crossover with the type of care offered in the community as well as intermediate care. You are, in effect, working in the patient's home, with structured care plans that will last years, rather than the sometimes fleeting moments shared with patients in other settings. You are there for daily medications, to make sure food is served on time, rooms and beds are cleaned, families are accommodated for and, in times such as during the COVID-19 pandemic, precautions are taken to ensure the safety of the residents.

You are often dealing with sick and ailing people, mostly elderly, who have perhaps lost their ability to live independently and require round-the-clock care. There are extreme joys to be found in this work, dealing with patients with incredible life stories who you will come to know as family. To play games or help with arts and crafts and share stories, there are many ways in which this setting differs from the care you can provide as a nurse elsewhere. You will equally encounter many times when relatives will show a deep appreciation for your work in helping their family member to live as best as they can under the circumstances.

On the other hand, consider this work to be intense, with real challenges over short staffing, long hours, and in some cases there are patients or families who will challenge the level of care they receive, making it daunting to deal with some residents. This can be the case in many other lines of nursing work too, but in a care facility, other staff and management should be on hand to help.

There are many nurses who will be inspired to enter this profession because they have first-hand knowledge of the care a relative received and wish to pass that on to others. There is no doubt it is a very necessary area of the health and care system, helping to look after patients in a more independent manner and to lessen the impact on numbers in the hospital.

Intermediate Care

Intermediate care is also designed to relieve the pressure on hospitals, while at the same time affording patients a better sense of independence as they cope with a variety of health issues.

As a free service to patients, it can take place in acute or community hospitals, residential care homes and at the individual's home, where patients are supported by intermediate care staff in ways to prevent them from needing other hospital stays or to support their follow-up care.

This is a short-term service, but it is vital to help patients' recovery. It can also bring you, as a nurse, into contact with other health professionals, such as occupational therapists, physiotherapists and speech and language therapists, as well as staff in care homes.

Stacey Finlay registered as a nurse in 2017 and began her career in an intermediate care unit within a private nursing home. Stacey has worked in intermediate care even before she decided to embark on her nursing degree, and now, a unit sister/manager, Stacey still loves her job despite the many challenges this sector regularly faces.

I found whilst studying that my favourite area of practice and population to look after was older people. I found this specialty much more interesting than areas that focus on particular body systems. Generally in life, I have very eclectic tastes, and career-wise I'm no different. I like and thrive on variety, and geriatrics brings that in droves! With the added benefit of working with a very interesting patient group and a focus on trying to help people live as well as possible for as long as possible, I believe geriatrics really is the specialty for me.

Whilst Stacey enjoyed her hospital-based placements as a student, she felt like there was something missing.

I always had this feeling that the patients I was seeing in hospital, I was seeing too late. They were already unwell a lot of the time. I felt that working in a setting where I could work with older people whilst they were more upstream than downstream would be what I would find most rewarding and where my input could have the most benefit. As I was already familiar with intermediate care and enjoyed my time there, I decided that once registered, I would start my nursing career in this area, and over four years later, I'm still here. Only now I'm the unit sister instead of staff nurse.

In Stacey's role as a nurse in the intermediate care unit, she helps to provide short-term rehabilitation for older people following an acute admission for any reason that has caused their mobility to deteriorate below their baseline.

We don't just focus on fixing the acute problem, we also look at the person as a whole and try to establish why they ended up in a hospital in the first place and if there is a possibility that a similar admission could reoccur and if there is anything else we could do to improve quality of life. We look at everything from their medicines to their shoes!

Selling Points of Intermediate Care

The other major selling point I found with geriatrics was the multidisciplinary nature of the specialty. All members of the team are involved in weekly multidisciplinary meetings about the patients, and everyone has an equally valued input. This equality and the setting in itself allows nurses to be more autonomous in our practice.

Career Development in Intermediate Care

I have completed postgraduate diplomas in both advanced practice and care of the elderly and have also completed a short course in palliative and end-of-life care in my role. I use my newfound skills, particularly when there is no medical staff in the building. I would often be asked to assess patients who may be showing signs of illness. I can request investigations such as bloods, form a diagnosis and plan for review by medical staff when it is most appropriate for the patient.

Tips for Choosing a Career in Intermediate Care

My first tip for new nurses considering this area – don't listen to those that tell you that you must start your career on an acute ward, as you will 'lose your skills'. This was something I was told as a student every time I said where I planned to start my career. All of the misconceptions are completely untrue. Each area requires different skills, but when you look at essential nursing and assessment skills, I use them constantly.

Nurse Bank or Agency Work

Many of the roles we've discussed will have set hours and rotas, generally spelled out well in advance. However, what if you desire more flexibility, or simply the ability to pick and choose your days, hours or place of work? This is where the nurse bank or agency work comes in. Effectively, this is freelance work, with no further commitment than the shift or shifts you agree to take on. While it is open to people who have full-time or part-time jobs elsewhere or those who would like the extra hours and money, the nurse bank or agency work can be a full-time pursuit if it works for the individual.

Of course there are some entry requirements. You may need six to 12 months experience working as a registered nurse before you can confidently take on a role with an agency or the nurse bank. This is purely because you will need to get certain skills signed off that would be useful while working with the agency/bank, i.e. intravenous drug administration, insertion of cannulas, catheter insertion, etc.

For those who take on nurse bank/agency shifts outside of their normal working hours, be sure that this is a commitment you can manage. You will hear a lot about nurse burnout, and we will discuss this later in the book. While the extra money can be tempting, make sure that you keep a balance and look after yourself as well. You know that saying, 'if you can't look after yourself how do you expect to look after sick patients'?

But what is the nurse bank/agency?

NURSE BANK

The nurse bank is generally used to plug gaps in rotas and to call upon staff in emergency situations where extra cover is required. It is usually associated with and managed by a particular trust who will issue appeals, often by text message, to let registered nurses know there are shifts available. Nurse bank work tends to operate at an enhanced payment rate, with some weekend and overnight shifts commanding an even higher fee.

AGENCY

Agency work is similar to the nurse bank but operates through a private sector company. It also has an enhanced fee, and as a registered nurse, you can work for the National Health Service (NHS) and also take on agency work around your normal hours. There are sometimes further requirements to research, such as you may not be able to take on shifts within your own health trust.

I love being on the nurse bank, I can take on a few more shifts whenever I need some extra money for things like holidays or Christmas.

(EMMETT, STAFF NURSE IN A FULL-TIME POST AND A REGULAR ON THE NURSE BANK)

Working for the agency offers me so much flexibility. I have two small children, so trying to manage my time around my husband's shifts and my own was a nightmare when I had a permanent post. Now, I can pick and choose when I want to work, so if the weather is nice one day…and let's face it, in Wales it's rarely sunny… I can choose not to work and make the most of the sunshine with my children and just take on a shift another day.

(OLGA, AGENCY WORKER)

Both the nurse bank and agency work can have its advantages to many, but like every job, there are also some things that aren't great. Take a look below at some of the pros, cons and my useful tips for your working life on the nurse bank or with an agency.

Pros

- You can earn more money than the normal standard rate you would get with a permanent post in a trust. Some trusts offer a higher hourly rate for bank nurses, and it is commonly known that agency workers do get paid more per hour than trust staff.
- You can do shifts in multiple different areas that aren't your usual place of work, meaning you can gain numerous new skills and experience you may not be exposed to in a permanent post.
- There are pretty much shifts available every day and at any time, so you can choose your own work schedule and be flexible with your hours.
- Usually, the area you choose to take a bank/agency shift is very understaffed and therefore appreciative of your help, meaning you get the good vibes from colleagues that you are making a difference just by being there and helping them out.

Cons

- Despite the shortages of nurses and the ever-growing need for shifts to be filled, you may find it difficult navigating these shifts around your full-time work, especially as the nurse bank/agency shifts may be in areas you don't like, can't travel to or don't have the experience or expertise for. There is no guarantee you will get a shift at a time and date that suits you in an area you want to work in.

- You may not have access to certain things on shift, i.e. computer login, keys for the drug rooms, passes for certain machines and access through doors of different departments, etc.
- You may not be familiar with the area you are working in, meaning it may take you longer doing specific tasks as you try to work out where everything is and what everyone's role is in this particular area.
- On some occasions, there is a risk that you may agree to a certain shift only to be moved last minute to another area in greater need.

Tips

- Say hello to everyone and introduce yourself. If you haven't done a shift like this before or this is a new area for you, then let the people you are working with know so it's not a surprise if you ask for help or advice. Introducing yourself to someone is a way of opening up a relationship with them you may need to call upon later in your shift.
- Be clear about your skills and competencies. For example, if you aren't yet signed off on cannulations, then tell someone this. I always found it useful when starting out to tell another nurse, *'Hi there, my patient needs a male catheter insertion and I haven't yet completed this skill. Could I do a task for you and in turn could you do this for me or supervise me while I attempt if the patient is consenting?'* This shows you are willing to work and not passing your jobs off onto the other staff who have their own workload.
- Make a 'to do' list and plan out your day after handover so you don't miss anything and you know what needs to happen and when.
- Ask the permanent staff questions. This doesn't have to be with another registered nurse but can be catering staff, nursing assistants and even students. Everyone will have their own experience, and you never know what little nuggets of gold you find out that will help you to have a successful shift.

Working Abroad

They say nursing is a passport to the world, and it truly is, but what if your life-long dream post-registration is to emigrate and start your career in another country? Before you pack your bags, your PIN and of course this book and set off into the sunset, there are a few things you might like to consider. Let's take a look at Box 2.1.

BOX 2.1 ■ Things to Consider

- Are you qualifications transferable? What is nursing like in this country, and how does it differ from where you trained?
- Will you need to complete any extra qualifications to work as a nurse in your chosen destination?
- If this will be your first job, will your employer support you, and will you have the opportunity to have a preceptorship period?
- What skills do you need for your chosen job, and do you have these?
- What is the salary like in this country? Do you need to consider exchange rates? How much will it cost to visit home?
- Do you need a work visa?
- Do you speak the language?

Continued

> **BOX 2.1 ■ Things to Consider—cont'd**
>
> ■ What are the hours of work in this country for nurses?
> ■ Where will you live? Do you need a driver's licence?
> ■ Do you need to pay for and apply to be put onto the nursing register in this country?

Ensuring that you meet the requirements to nurse in your chosen country is one thing; however, keep in mind that if you wish to retain a United Kingdom (UK) registration to return to, you will have to complete revalidation every three years and pay your annual Nursing and Midwifery Council (NMC) retention fee. The NMC also advises that you register with the appropriate regulator wherever it is that you are working. It is also worth researching what the best trade union is to join, as, for example, the Royal College of Nursing (RCN) is only a trade union in the UK, Channel Islands and the Isle of Man and cannot offer formal advice or representation for matters in the host country.

An important thing to consider is whether your UK qualification is transferable to the country you wish to work in, or do you need to complete additional exams or assessments to gain the requirements for the job you are applying for.

The key advice for considering nursing abroad is do your research.

I moved to Australia to live out my dream of being a nurse and to go surfing and sunbathing every day. It was so time consuming getting everything organised and making sure I had ticked all the boxes, but in the end, I am so happy with my decision to move abroad. Nursing is so different here, but I love this lifestyle, I don't see myself giving up on the sunshine here for the rain back home anytime soon

(JOSIE, A NURSE WHO MOVED TO AUSTRALIA)

Another way of working abroad is through humanitarian efforts and charity. This could be a career path or volunteering, with international development and relief organisations making regular appeals for nurses to help in poorer regions of the world or following disasters. You could work directly for the United Nations through a number of their agencies, such as the United Nations Children's Fund (Unicef) or the World Food Programme (WFP). In these roles, you could encounter wars, famine and extreme hardships. Such a testing environment can bring satisfaction that your work is making a difference to people in great need; however, also consider the mental and physical strains and challenges that it will pose to a nurse under these circumstances.

Working in the Military

This can be an exciting career for some with the chance to train in far-off lands and to operate as a nurse in unique circumstances. From military exercises to the battlefield, this is a different setting to the regular hospital ward or anything you could taste from your placements. It goes without saying that to work in the military you must first buy into the added element of risk and danger. Army medics have been on the frontline and lost their lives while trying to save others.

Working in the military is emergency medicine at its most raw. Many of today's modern nursing techniques were honed through helping soldiers in tents during world wars. Their injuries and the resources available meant many nurses had to use what they could, and do what they could, for patients who were suffering in ways few can imagine. Florence Nightingale made her name because of her actions during the Crimean War. History tells us that nurses play a vital role during times of conflict; perhaps this could be your calling too?

It is a field in which our profession has acted with distinction for many generations. But it is not to be entered into lightly.

Specialist Nursing

Nurse specialists are role models and leaders in improving nursing practice and the delivery of patient care. They are experts in their field and admired by all members of the nursing family. Nurse specialists can work in and out of hospital settings and in a variety of roles. They can give advice on care, whilst also providing it. They are educators, researchers and clinicians who use their skills and expertise to benefit the patients and the profession. They gain their knowledge through a combination of work-based experience and further education and training. Take a look at Box 2.2 for some nurse specialist roles.

BOX 2.2 ■ Career Opportunities for Specialist Nurses

- Nurse anaesthetist; helps to provide anaesthesia for patients undergoing surgery and assists looking after them during the operation.
- Nurse educator; training, educating, and shaping nurses of the future.
- Nurse practitioner; advanced nurse who can collaborate with a doctor to provide care or run their own clinics.
- Nurse researcher; gathering evidence used to improve patient care delivery

---

These are jobs for which you will need further training and time experience before you can apply for them, but you can begin to think about these roles from the moment you register. If there is an area you are particularly interested in, it might be worth asking a nurse specialist who works in that area what their job entails and what qualifications they needed to obtain this role so you can begin to think about your future.

Choosing Where to Work

People often say, 'next to the patient is where a nurse should be', but this isn't always the case. Nurses do not always need to work in patient-facing roles to make an impact. Consider those, such as the chief nursing officer, who work at a policy and strategic level, engaging with other health leaders to influence change on the ground. Nurse lecturers see students, not patients (although some may still practice), and have a major impact on the lives of prospective nurses who in turn will go on to use the knowledge and experience they've gained to improve the health of others. Ultimately, at every level, if you work in healthcare, you are working for the betterment of the patient, whether you have direct contact with them or not.

When choosing where you want to work, there are a number of things you will need to consider:

- What area of nursing am I attracted to?
- Can I be flexible or do I need a job that has stable hours?
- Do I work better alone or would I benefit from regular colleague interaction?
- Do I get stressed easily or thrive under pressure?
- Are there some areas that I will need to avoid due to emotional triggers?
- Is part-time or full-time most suitable?
- What experience do I already have and will this benefit me in certain roles?
- What parts of nursing do I enjoy and what areas do I not?
- Where do I see my career going long-term?
- Do I already have plans for my future? What job would assist in achieving this?
- Will I work at home or abroad?
- Do I need to travel to the role I am considering applying for and how will this work out in reality?

Let's make a list of your top three jobs or areas you would like to work in.

1. _____

2. _____

3. _____

Now let's take each job individually and make a pros and cons list for each:

Job One:

_____

_____

Pros

_____

_____

_____

_____

_____

_____

_____

_____

Cons

_____

_____

_____

_____

_____

_____

_____

_____

_____

_____

_____

Job Two:

_____

_____

Pros

_____

_____

_____

_____

_____

_____

_____

_____

_____

_____

Cons

_____

_____

_____

_____

_____

_____

_____

_____

_____

_____

_____

_____

Job Three:

_____

_____

Pros

_____

_____

_____

_____

_____

_____

_____

_____

_____

Cons

_____

_____

_____

_____

_____

_____

_____

_____

_____

_____

Now you have considered the pros and cons of each job, take a look at them again. Can you narrow it down to two?

Take each of these and figure out what you need to actually start working there and make a list of what you will do to achieve this.

Job One:

_____

_____

What Do I Need to Work Here?

_____

_____

_____

_____

_____

_____

_____

How Will I Achieve This?

_____

_____

_____

_____

_____

_____

_____

_____

_____

_____

_____

Job Two:

_____

_____

What Do I Need to Work Here?

_____

_____

_____

_____

_____

_____

_____

_____

_____

_____

_____

How Will I Achieve This?

_____

_____

_____

_____

_____

_____

_____

_____

_____

_____

_____

It can be difficult to plan your career; however, you have had these dilemmas before. In choosing which GCSEs to study, to apply for nursing, to reach for a guidebook such as this, you have spent years yearning for information and making decisions that have led you to this point. You have probably sought advice along the way; be sure to call upon that again now.

Whatever line of work in nursing you go for, it doesn't have to be a forever job. New opportunities will arise, team dynamics can change over time that makes you wish for a change; or, perhaps you develop a desire to travel and experience new things that breach your comfort zone. Maybe you fall in love with a new discipline or something prompts you to follow a different path. As we have discussed, there are many avenues open to you in this incredible career, and change is rarely easy. Whatever you choose, just remember why you started.

CHAPTER 3

How to Land the Job!

Ok, so it's that time. The qualification is in the bag and you are set for a nursing career. First of all, well done reaching this point, even if the next stage can feel daunting. Allow yourself a moment to revel in that achievement, because now the real work starts. But how exactly do you go from being the student on the ward to the full-fledged nurse with that extra level of responsibility?

Good news. You're not the first to apply, and there are many well-trodden paths to follow. Where you start in your nursing career can come down to many factors, which we will explore, but like many jobs, it will most likely involve an application, an interview, hours of nail biting, then either acceptance or – and we will examine how it is not the end of the world – a dreaded rejection.

One thing we can all be sure of: the world needs nurses. If the job market looks challenging, know from the outset that you may deviate during your career wildly from post to post, discipline to discipline. You could start in a 100-miles-per-hour ward, with emergencies left, right and centre, then take up a post in research, for instance, where the role is still important but without such frantic moments. Or you may enter lecturing, or find that your new role takes you travelling, in the community or even to a battlefield.

What I mean is that your first job doesn't have to be the dream job. That may need work and time to reach. The ideal area for your skills and ambitions may also not be obvious yet, so whatever your first steps become, allow yourself to enjoy the journey and give yourself space and time to grow.

But where do I look for a job?

The following advice applies whether this is your first role or if you have reached a stage where you wish for a change. In the case of the former, your university or course should be a firm starting place, as they will have an established resource of other guidebooks and career advisors who are on hand to chat through your options. Be open with advisors about your experience and your ambitions. If they do not know a direct route, they should be able to advise ways in which you can shape your career ahead to reach that end goal. There may also be established connections with local health trusts or organisations which are looking for new nurses but have not advertised their roles widely. If you don't ask, you may not know!

The Internet

It's the 2020s, and the internet is most likely where you will find out about new opportunities and will act as your means to apply for them. From central bodies to local trusts and groups, pretty much every organisation looking for a nurse will post the role to their website. Most will have a dedicated 'work for us' type area or a news alert about fresh advertisements. If they have nothing available, there may be a form which you can use to subscribe to e-mails about their next recruitment run. Hopefully, they will explain the demands and job criteria clearly, but if they do not, this should be available, so contact them to ask.

Chances are the website will link to the organisation's social media offerings which, in this day and age, most will have. Often, job advertisements will appear on the likes of Facebook, Twitter and Instagram containing links to where you can apply. Sometimes these posts will show that they have been shared many times, or plenty of people have commented linking the post to their contacts. Do not let that put you off. Be proud of your achievements and never assume that a post which seems to have a lot of interest will translate into a million applications. Even if it does, believe in yourself and give it a shot if it is something you want.

Websites such as www.jobs.nhs.uk or www.nhsjobs.com could be good starting places, as they allow you to search a broad spectrum of roles to get an idea of what is out there.

If the process is daunting, many recruitment websites will allow you to filter a search, making the internet possibly your easiest method of tailoring a job hunt. With the click of a button, you can hone in on your desired location, or expand the field to search for jobs within a set distance. The salary or type of work could come next, with other options about whether the job is permanent or temporary, full-time or part-time. Play about with these fields to see if there are enticing opportunities which meet your criteria. However, also broaden your search and think outside the box. Maybe that dream position is a mile or two outside your set parameters and you could be overlooking it. Or what if there is a job title which seems a little left-field at first for your desires but when you actually read the description, the at-first unattractive title appears to be a role you get excited about.

I looked at my trust's recruitment page and seen a job in haematology nursing. At first, I disregarded this job as I thought, 'well you won't be qualified enough for that type of nursing yet.' As I scrolled through the page, nothing else stood out to me. I went back and looked at the haematology job and found they were accepting newly registered nurses! I applied and here I am five years later doing my specialist training to be a haemophilia nurse. My advice is, put your hat in the ring, you never know what will come of it.

(Haematology nurse Anna)

Publications

Both official nursing publications and the media are prime target areas for recruiters, as they will reach a wide audience. You may even see that the recruitment graphic design team have used the same jazzy advert online as they do in print.

You should check local and national newspapers, as they will usually have a job section. Some will have it on certain days of the week, while others will have a fixed set of pages every day. The *Nursing Standard* and *Nursing Times* are good examples of print editions which know their audience and should be an obvious port for your job-hunting mind to call on.

READ ALL ABOUT IT, READ ALL ABOUT IT, NURSES WANTED

Recruitment Events

Yes, it is not all about the pens, post-it notes and, if you are lucky with your choice of fair, a slice of free pizza. Job events and conferences for nurses are a useful resource when planning your first or next move. You could be inspired by something you had not previously considered, or get the chance, face-to-face, to ask people who have the job you want how they got there and their advice on how you can follow. Take leaflets, bring your friends and have an open mind.

And remember: if nothing comes of it, use those free pens to write that perfect application when the time is right!

> In 2015, I attended the Royal College of Nursing's (RCN) annual Congress. I was a final-year student at the time and still a few months to go in my degree, but I met a prospective employer at this event and talked them through my experience and what type of nursing I wanted to pursue. A few minutes later we had set up my application and interview right there on the spot. They explained to me the various opportunities they had, we talked about hours, perks of the employer, and they even gave me advice for my interview. It's now a few years later and I am gearing up to attend the same event as a representative for the same employer who was so kind and patient with me all those years ago. I hope to see some of you there.
>
> **(Staff Nurse Tim)**

Word of Mouth

Think back to any jobs you had before you set off on this magical path to nursing. How did you hear about them? For many, it will have been a nod or a share of information from someone else who knew about an opening, or somewhere that was hiring and thought it was worth you knowing too. Think people-first and, in this instance, remind your friends and family you are on the lookout for opportunities and hope they can report back with news on the grapevine. If you have contacts in the area you want to work in, savour that connection and use it to your advantage for hints and tips.

This does not mean that you should canvass for a job or expect to be advantaged by some form of insider information, but quite often it will be someone else who notices a job listing and mentions, 'did you see that job advert…' or 'I think they might be looking for a nurse to fill X role' that will spark your interest.

Never fear contacting managers or fellow nurses about their job area and what you would need to position yourself well for success. Think a number of career stages ahead if you are ambitious and question why they were successful and how you can be too. Be polite and inquisitive. Every nurse was you once, and someday you could be the one giving out the career advice.

The Application

The empty boxes stare back, waiting to be filled. Oh, the dread!

First things first, get yourself together, this is your first impression. The person reading it does not know you, how amazing you are or what you want. Yet.

That does not mean you can play make-believe like you are some form of nurse Avenger and exaggerate your skills to superhero level… Let me say this early: do not lie on your application. Honesty is the best policy.

The following pieces of advice may not be relevant for your next application, but they are good things to constantly think about and keep fresh.

DECLARATIONS

This is so important that it needs to trump the other topics. If you have a disability, do not fear declaring it in the application. Under equality legislation, employers must not discriminate on the grounds of disability, which can of course come in many forms. Under the Equality Act 2010, which applies in Great Britain, a person with a disability must be interviewed if they meet the minimum job requirements.

There are protections too in terms of race, gender, religious belief, pregnancy and maternity, marriage and civil partnerships. Similar legislation exists in Northern Ireland and, if the candidate is successful, there are legal obligations on employers to meet access and support needs.

Everyone has the right to apply for a job and to feel supported and protected by it. You will notice in searching for jobs that many employers will also stipulate that they encourage applications from particular groups of people. There is an increasing awareness of the benefits of a diverse workforce, and these legal protections will hopefully encourage more people to stand up for their rights.

THE CURRICULUM VITAE

Haven't written a curriculum vitae (CV) before? Don't know what it is?

Well, let this be the time you start one. A CV is a personal greatest hits selection. Your own 'Now that's what I call a good nurse' hit list which at a glance can tell employers whether or not this candidate whose full application is before them is worthy of the job.

It can be the make or break and potentially, depending on how they review your application, could be the first thing they decide to read. So it is important to get it right.

There are countless resources online about how to write a good CV (or a resume, to coin the American phrase if it opens up more search options), so this will be a short introduction, but the important thing is to be truthful yet sell yourself.

List your educational attainments, with dates, and your previous employment experience as necessary. For people who enter nursing after having had a different type of career, include your past jobs and sell the fact that these have built your skills and character alongside the nursing qualification that brings you to this point.

When writing the CV, be professional, use sensible fonts (as tempting as Comic Sans can be) and a neat layout. Most writing software programmes will even have a CV template if it helps you get started on this.

Under your previous work, include relevant duties which tailor your CV to the job you are applying for. Did you have responsibility for an important aspect of the work or lead a team? Did your role require proficiency with software or numbers? Did you deal with the public or other stakeholders?

Even if it does not feel like a job which sells yourself as a nurse, there can be elements that you can enhance to show that you have a broader skillset than just your qualification.

Important too – do not overwrite and keep the whole CV to about two A4 pages long. Keep your sentences succinct and use professional words to sell your experience. You will have opportunities elsewhere to delve into the courses, jobs and interests you list here.

Remember to always update your CV and think of how you can change it to suit the next job you apply for.

Another safety net piece of advice to offer is asking someone you trust to read it. Check for typos and see if they remember relevant experience you forgot to mention.

A CV may help you remember skills you can go on to outline in the application or discuss at the interview, but if you go through this process and feel your CV is inadequate or that it becomes a thoroughly depressing endeavour, seek advice and help over how to sell the things you have done or what your next step should be to add to the CV things which are currently lacking.

Exercise: List here three things you think you should include in your CV and three things you think you should avoid.

Things to add to my CV	Things I should avoid on my CV
E.g. Training I have completed which is relevant to this new role	E.g. Lying or exaggerating my skills and abilities
1	1
2	2
3	3

To help you further, I have included at the end of this chapter a blank template of a CV for you to complete. This may or may not be what your CV will look like in practice, but it will give you some hints and tips to get you started.

A COVER LETTER

This is different from a CV and may not be required by every employer, so always check what they need.

Generally, it is a personal statement, an opportunity for you to sell yourself and delve deeper into the elements listed on your CV, but with more specific reference to why you are the right candidate for this job.

There is more scope here for descriptive language and a chance for you to cite a piece of experience from your CV and discuss what your position involved and how/why that experience means you are the best person for the job. It is also an opening for you to go into more detail as a newly registered nurse about your course or degree and what you did in extracurricular terms to better yourself.

For instance, did you take part in societies, magazines, union activity, anything else which sets you apart and shows your motivation? These may seem trivial when applying for a big, serious job, but remember they can demonstrate a hard work ethic, dedication, your ability to work with teams and generate fresh thinking. Exactly the type of person this employer might want to be part of their team alongside the necessary qualification.

Always be positive (but not arrogant), and do not focus on things you 'do not have', but discuss what you offer and why you believe this job needs you to fill it.

THE BOXES

OK, so we have the CV and the cover letter/personal statement, whatever they might call it. Depending on the job, there may also be a section we can only really refer to as 'the boxes' because they can involve pretty much anything. You know the types of questions: 'Why do you believe you are the best candidate?' or a prompting statement such as: 'Demonstrate how you meet the desired level of experience.'

The first piece of advice: for this type of question, take it in and slowly walk away from the application. Yes, close it and walk away. This is your time to shine and:

A. You do not want to hit that submit button by accident if it looms where your mouse can click it.
B. You need space to see your answer, not a cramped box you need to scroll about in.
C. This is another chance to ask someone to check your work and whether it can be improved.

So, go old-school and use a pen and paper, or make a note on your phone, maybe even a crisp clean white page in Word. Put the question at the top and give yourself time to think it through, maybe even bullet point a few key topics you want to touch on so you don't forget.

This allows you to draft until your heart is content and make adjustments over time to get it right.

Take the word count for the boxes seriously. There will be ways to fill it, but also be conscious of how it looks if you barely take up space in a box when you had the room to write an essay. There is a healthy middle to be found between waffling on and not really answering the question.

To start, think about what they are asking for. The wording may have been chosen deliberately, one would assume, to filter out candidates they are not looking for and phrased in a way that will allow you to explore why you meet their criteria and should make the next stage of the process.

There should be a lengthy job description somewhere, outlining the essential and desired criteria. Some things are essential, such as a qualification level, and are possibly non-negotiable when it comes to the employer considering candidates. Think carefully if it is worth your having a go if you feel you fall well short of this. Desirable criteria can be more open-ended and range from experience levels to whether or not you can use certain software. To list something as desirable implies there could be some wriggle room if you do not meet these criteria, but you would be expected to demonstrate ways in which you meet a lot of it. Do you speak another language and the criteria ask for it? Well, make sure it is included. Or, for example, you may be asked if you have a valid driving licence. If you don't, but are currently working towards it, do not leave this section blank. Instead, answer the question with something like this:

> *I do not yet currently hold a valid driving licence; however, I am in the process of achieving this. I have been delayed in doing so due to the COVID-19 pandemic but hope to meet this criteria in the very near future* (but don't lie if you are not actively trying to achieve your driving licence).

Keep in mind, there are unlikely to be any extra points for getting an application in early, so unless the deadline is already bearing down on you, take some time to re-read your answers and invite others to give their thoughts on how you have structured things, as well as checking for the odd typo which anyone can be guilty of.

REFERENCES

If the job asks for a reference, make yours a good one. This does not mean you get your mum or your best friend to write up a glowing report on why you are brilliant, but it is a professional endorsement from someone whose contribution to the application process could be invaluable when jobs are decided on the narrowest of margins. Think about past employers, places where you did placements during your course, or your course lecturers. Who has the gravitas and knowledge of your skillset to write with authority about what you will bring to the position you are applying for? This does not have to be a dissertation-length biography, but a letter that gives enough detail for the reader to take notice.

The short list and the interview

Ok, it's happening. Stay calm. I repeat, don't panic.

You have bossed round one. Bank that good energy, as things are about to get serious.

You have heard the Oscar speech many times – it was lovely just to be nominated… well, it really is nice to be shortlisted.

Out of presumably many candidates, you have got through the first difficult stage and almost like the X-Factor, you are ready to set off to the judges' houses.

Shortlisting usually means the next stage is the interview. So, let's prepare.

Preparing for the interview worksheet

PREPARING FOR THE INTERVIEW

The single most important thing before we work out what your answers should be is making sure you know when and where the interview is and that you can guarantee you will make it in good time. If you have other commitments, such as childcare, approach the employer and discuss if you require alternative arrangements to be made. If distance is an issue, there has been a trend, particularly during the pandemic, for interviews to be conducted online. It may not always be possible, but try to suss out your options early so it does not become last-minute stress.

Equally, you need to appear professional. A smart business outfit or suit is the order of the day for a nurse interview, regardless of whether the job will require you to scrub up rather than tie on. Make sure you know what you will wear and that it fits you. Seek the advice of others if you are unsure about your choice; again, the last thing you want is an eleventh-hour dash to the shops.

With a prepared mind comes a clear one to think about what you will say when you enter the room.

It is likely that your interview will follow a traditional format. Two, maybe three people on a panel, all taking turns to ask questions, all writing down notes which will be reflected on afterwards to score each candidate. They may ask for a presentation. Some jobs will also have an element where they bring in a group of candidates to work together then present something to the panel.

Some questions are predictable, give or take, and some others are not. So let's focus first on those you can fairly guarantee will come up, as you can make notes in advance. Think of these as pointers to which your answers can be used elsewhere if they do not come up word-for-word.

- Welcome to the interview, why do you want the job?
- Tell us how your experience relates to this role?
- What is your understanding of our organisation?
- Tell us about times you have worked under pressure?

Take a look at the end of this chapter. We have included these questions for you to write down some of your thoughts to help you get started.

Make notes, long-form first, then bullet points, about your experience, times when you were challenged, moments when you worked as a team, or led a group of people, occasions when you had arguments but found a resolution. What was it like in your placement? Did you see things you believe could change for the better in health care, in case they ask a question along those lines? What trends do you see appearing in nursing practice that will become influential in the future?

Bring these notes with you on the day in the most succinct form you can make them. They will be useful to scan through, and some panels will allow you to use them in the interview itself in case you lose your train of thought, but always check this out in advance.

Think of loads of examples from your experience. Big and small, serious and tedious. It can be a dangerous game to second-guess the questions and only prepare examples for them. Have examples in your back pocket which you can spring on the panel if the moment is nigh.

List words, too, which are the type of buzzwords which score well in interviews: organisational skills, communication and time management. Yes, they are cringe-worthy terms which rarely come up in day-to-day life, but an interview is not like a normal everyday-life conversation. It is a formal session to test if you 'get' what this job is about and whether you fit the bill.

Interviewers will often end the interview with a 'do you have any questions for us' question. This may not be scored, but it is something which can leave a final impression before you disappear hurriedly out the door. Try to think about something specific to the role or the employer other than 'when will I hear the result,' even if that is all you want to know.

Here are some questions you may ask:

- Throughout my research and preparation for this interview I came across a publication on how preceptorship enhances the experience of the newly registered nurse. Can you tell me if this job will include a preceptorship programme?
- I was wondering if your area has an induction programme for new recruits like myself, if successful?

MANAGING THE INTERVIEW

Be early, be smartly dressed, and be prepared.

And when we say smartly dressed, this means avoid distractions for the panel. Be formal, but be yourself; only you can judge what this means. This book is not meant to be a bible for how you should look and act, but just consider how excited the panel will be to meet you after that wonderful impression you made in the application. Now, here you are, walking into the room. What will they make of how you appear?

It almost goes without saying, a job interview is one of the most nerve-wracking things you can go through, particularly if it is for a position you desperately want. There can be real pressure on what it means for your future success or otherwise, and despite the best advice in the world about staying calm and relaxed, there is a lot at stake, and it can affect people in different ways.

A few pieces of advice, though, can help to ease that.

- When you are in the interview, pace yourself, both in speech and mind.
- Greet the panel and settle into the chair.
- Smile – it always helps.
- Take a sip of water, take your time. It is easy to feel your heart race and believe your words need to catch up.
- Take a deep breath and compose your opening remarks.
- Talk slower if it helps to structure your thoughts. The panel will likely be writing as you are talking, so you want to make sure they can take in your important points.
- If you need to joke about feeling nervous, say it. Give yourself the best chance to push past that tension rather than bottling it up and regretting how you handled the moment.

Often the first question will be general, something like why you want the job or believe you are the best candidate.

This is as straightforward a question as you could imagine and gives you the chance to talk at length about your strengths. Do not be afraid to pause and collect your thoughts during this, especially if you feel nervous. It can be the case that with the first question out of the way you can settle into the process and let the adrenaline take its place.

If questions follow which are confusing in how they are worded or you do not instantly know what to say, ask for them to be repeated or clarify with the panel so you know what they are getting at. It will save them having to interject if your answer goes down the wrong path, but it may be that this extra second or two allows your mind to grab hold of the relevant example or point you wish to use.

What If I Don't Get the Job?

There is no papering over how disappointing a moment this can be, and it may cause you to feel down or struggle to work out the repercussions of not getting the job.

It is a test of character, and one can only recommend surrounding yourself with friends and family to get their support and advice on the next steps.

As a newly registered nurse, this can be a hard rejection to take as you are setting off on an exciting career only to have it seemingly halted in front of you.

Of course, this simply is not the case. Your qualification speaks for itself and there will be other opportunities out there. The United Kingdom (UK) and the world need more nurses, there is a shortage of our skills. The headlines constantly talk of the country 'crying out for new nurses,' so once your own tears subside, it is time to get back to work. We are in this together.

You may never find this out, but fine margins may have meant that you did not get the job this time. It may not have been your shortcomings, rather that another candidate was just that little bit further in front.

So, always ask for feedback. The worst that can come of this is that you learn some lessons from your interview performance or the skills you need to nail the job down the next time.

Your nursing career will be based on constantly learning lessons, from the lecture hall to the challenging moments in dealing with a sick patient. We are all human, and it is often how we react to low moments that make us stronger.

It may not have been for you, but it could be the next time.

To paraphrase President John F. Kennedy – nurses do things not because they are easy, but because they are hard.

Below you will find some prompts to help you complete your CV. This may or may not be what your final CV will look like but it will help on your way to getting started.

Welcome to the interview, why do you want the job?

List four reasons why you want the job you are applying for…

1. ....
....
....

2. ....
....
....

3. ....
....
....

4. ....
....
....

Tell us how your experience relates to this role

Think about what skills/ achievements you have that would help you in this new role? Think about placement experience, part-time jobs you've had, any volunteer work you have done. What about your life before nursing, can you draw on that experience? Think of three…

1. ....
....
....

2. ....
....
....

3. ....
....
....

What is your understanding of our organisation?

Do your research! Take a look online for information about the organisation you are applying for and find out at least three facts about them. This could be anything from their motto to a recent good news story about them.

1. ....
....
....

2. ....
....
....

3. ....
....
....

Tell us about times you have worked under pressure?

As a recent student nurse, you will have experience of working under pressure. This can be from busy placement days to managing a 4000-word essay while holding down a part-time job and taking care of your family. Think of times when you had a lot on your plate but you managed things well. Think of two…

1. ....
....
....

2. ....
....
....

Name:

Contact details

Address:

Email:

Telephone number:

A little bit about me…

Write a few short lines about who you are. If you are still a student waiting on your degree classification, then state, 'final year student nurse due to qualify in August, predicted grade 2:1'. Discuss attributes such as your work ethic or your passions for nursing; however, try to keep this short and concise and no more than 100 words.

....

....

....

....

....

My achievements and key skills

Here you want to include things that set you apart from other candidates. Have you ever volunteered for an organisation? How did this help your communication and personal development? Do you have a special skill you could talk about? Can you speak another language or have you completed a course that may help you in your new role? Talk about these things and keep this to about 150 words.

....

....

....

....

....

Work/placement experience

List your work/placement experience by telling the reader the dates you had this experience and where. Write a few lines on what you gained from this and how it has helped you develop your nursing skills. Do not list every placement you have had, just pick a select few which stand out. About 100 words for each section will do.

....

....

....

....

....

Education and qualifications

Here you want to list your education and qualifications. You may not have your degree classification yet, but put down your predicted grade and your years of study. Keep this short; you don't need to explain this section, simply list them.

....

....

....

....

....

Professional training and activities

Simply list any training you have completed that may be relevant to the role which you are applying for. For example, have you completed your intermediate life support at university? Have you been on a course about dementia care? Well, list these here just like you did above – no need to explain each activity.

....

....

....

....

....

References

Almost all job applications will require at least two references. These need to be professional individuals who are aware of your abilities. Still at university? Ask a lecturer. List their name and contact details as well as their job title. They don't need to complete the reference immediately, just when the prospective employer asks for it, but make sure you always have their consent to being your reference first.

....

....

....

....

....

CHAPTER 4

Preceptorship: Getting the Most Out of It

Today we live in an age of innovation when technology is advancing at a remarkable rate.

When once a computer took up a room, now it fits in the palm of your hand. When it once took weeks to send a message from England to Australia, now it takes seconds to connect to a video chat. Our society is changing and so too is nursing.

Nurses are no longer seen as 'the handmaiden', but as leaders who play vital roles in transforming, leading and coordinating care that is underpinned by compassion, evidence and has the person (or patient) at its core. With this, nurses are accountable for their acts and omissions. They must work autonomously and as equal partners in the wider multidisciplinary team in order to meet the rising demands of the public and the increase in patients with complex and challenging co-morbidities. Being a nurse is a massive undertaking, a role with great responsibility and of vital importance.

With that being said, nurses of today must be emotionally intelligent and resilient, but also able to recognise and respond to their own personal health and know when to access support.

But who do nurses get support from? Who helps you when you're the new nurse and it's your first day?

> *It's 2 am and even though the alarm has a few hours before it wakes me, here I am, bright-eyed and terrified. Yes, excited, but also scared about what's to come. What if I forget my training and someone is really sick and it's all on me? Who do I call for help when they're all busy elsewhere? It feels real now.*
>
> **(EMMA BYRNE, NEWLY REGISTERED NURSE - REMEMBERING WHAT IT WAS LIKE AHEAD OF HER FIRST DAY)**

This is where preceptorship comes in.

What Is Preceptorship?

The transition from student to staff nurse can be a daunting and frightening experience. One minute you're a student and the next you're an accountable practitioner. This period is known to be challenging, but with the help of an experienced and competent nurse acting as your point person and role model, this transition can be a lot smoother. The goal of the preceptor is to provide support, valuable teaching and learning experiences which assist in integrating new nurses into their area of practice.

I trained in Scotland, but my first job was in my hometown in Northern Ireland, so on top of the fear of being just qualified, the worry about never working in Northern Ireland's health care system gave me serious anxiety. On my first day, I was a basket of nerves, then I met Minnie, my preceptor. Minnie was so welcoming, understanding and reassuring. I knew then and there that I would be okay.

(STAFF NURSE BARBARA, FIRST JOB)

According to the Nursing and Midwifery Council (NMC) (2020) in their Principles for Preceptorship, although voluntary, it is recommended that all newly registered nurses, those returning to practice and nurses transferring from other countries outside of the UK should have a period of preceptorship, stating: 'Although voluntary, we know preceptorship helps newly registered professionals have the best possible start as a registered professional in the UK' (NMC, 2020).

The role of the preceptorship process is to provide support during the transition from student to registered nurse. Although the NMC highly encourage the implementation of a preceptorship programme, it isn't mandatory. Whereas, most National Health Service (NHS) trusts across the UK have developed specific preceptorship programmes to suit the needs of the new nurses and nursing associates they hire, many areas in the private sector still have not made the same move. Despite this, there is plenty of support and advice out there from nursing unions and the NMC itself.

Lynsey McLaughlin is a newly registered nurse working in the private sector who has been through a preceptorship programme.

I was the first-ever newly registered nurse in my hospital, so the programme was completely new. I was essentially the guinea pig. As a theatre nurse, we cover lots of different specialities, meaning there is a lot to learn. So the plan was to keep me in one area for a time then move me to another.

I was lucky and got a full-year preceptorship where I was supposed to be supernumerary. This didn't always happen, but I stood my ground and voiced my concerns. Most people understood and I generally felt supported. I took turns in learning the different roles - the scrub, the circulating nurse and lastly anaesthetics. Overall, a lot of people were keen to teach.

The only negative in the private sector was a lot of my colleagues came from different hospitals, so they were taught how to do certain things differently depending on where they worked. As a result, I was taught how to do things in multiple ways, which was frustrating sometimes, as everyone felt their approach was the best one.

Before long, I was able to pick up the methods I felt most comfortable with and created my own way of doing things. I'm now confident with most surgeries and feel having experienced a preceptorship programme allowed me the time to focus on the type of nurse I want to be and how I can achieve that. I still have a lot to learn but I am happy with my progress.

Later in this chapter, there will be an opportunity for you to write down some thoughts and feelings about your own preceptorship. For now, though, let's get back into discovering how this process might work or differ depending on your area of work.

In most cases, the process should include at least one to two weeks where you work as a supernumerary nurse in order to grasp the routine of your new area of work. This process may include:

- **Shadowing:** You follow your named preceptor (or other staff) around to get an idea of what is going on in your new area of work. This will help you feel like you are starting to fit in with the team and the environment and to build up enough confidence to engage in clinical tasks.
- **Engagement:** You begin to ask questions and take on some tasks, under supervision and with support. Yes, you've got your pin, but it's a different ball game now that you've registered. Try to make the most of the supervision while it's available.

At this stage, you will be given appropriately sized chunks of work to complete so that your preceptor can assess your skill levels and abilities before you're left to work independently.

During the supernumerary period it could be useful to ask for the opportunity to explore areas relevant to your scope of practice; for example, attending theatre to observe if you're a surgical nurse or sitting in on different clinics if you work in a primary care setting. This will help you to integrate theory into your practice.

Mylena registered a few months ago and now works as a practice nurse in her local GP surgery. During Mylena's first few months in her new role, she took the opportunity of being supernumerary to explore the different departments within the practice. Mylena worked with the district nurses one day, another afternoon she shadowed the community midwife, next she sat in on a sexual and reproductive health clinic, and even assisted the nurse practitioner in carrying out their duties. Mylena now has more experience and information about what services her surgery provides, how her role links with others, who to contact in certain circumstances and a broader insight into the dynamics of the workplace.

Use the space below to make a list of some areas you could explore. Tick them off one by one when you have completed them. Add the dates and the hours spent and something you learned during this experience. This will help to show your progress no matter how small, and as an added bonus, all of this can be used for your revalidation, which we will cover in Chapter 12.

Areas to explore in my new role:	Dates and amount of hours I spent in this area:	What I learned during this experience:	Completed:

The preceptorship process gives you the opportunity to get familiar with your new area of work, your colleagues, the routine and everything that goes into being a successful and effective nurse in this area. Make sure you use this time wisely and take full advantage of asking many questions, even if you believe them to be stupid – you're safer asking them than making a mistake. Be supervised in doing as many tasks as possible and getting to know what your role is and the kind of nurse you want to be.

One afternoon I was working with a nurse who had just registered and had recently joined our team. He was so lovely and helpful and asked if there was anything I needed assistance with. I was happy for the help as we were already short-staffed. I asked if he could set up the feed for one of our residents. He accepted and went to walk away, but came back to say: 'I am so sorry, but this may sound really stupid, and I am really embarrassed to ask, but when you say set up the feed, what do you mean?' …I never really thought about it before, as it was just common lingo in our home. I meant the patient's feed for their nasogastric tube, but to someone new it could have seemed like I wanted them to make the resident their dinner. He wasn't stupid at all for asking me. In fact, it got me thinking about the terms and abbreviations we use in this job. It's like a different language sometimes.
(CIARA McKENNA, NURSING HOME, SENIOR NURSE)

During your preceptorship period, you will be assessed in many areas. You and your preceptor should meet at regular stages to discuss your progress, achievements and areas you need to improve on. While you are being assessed, you may find it useful to ask for feedback, written or verbal, from other members of staff you have worked with. This may also give you the opportunity to give input and feedback about yourself, your work, your preceptor and the area you're working in. This information can be used towards area audits, for your preceptor's revalidation and your own (once again, this will be covered in more detail in Chapter 12, so keep reading).

Some areas have their own programme, which includes booklets that new nurses must complete with role-specific competencies. Other areas offer programmes that include training days and lectures. Whatever area you work in, the key element in preceptorship is individualised support provided in practice by the preceptor.

Preceptorship Timeframe

The NMC recommends that all new registrants should have some sort of formal preceptorship period which may vary depending on individual need. This means, on occasion, some new nurses may require an extended period of supervision and some may require less.

The usual time frame for completing a preceptorship is around six to 12 months. This doesn't mean you'll be supernumerary for this whole period. What this means is that you'll have to be able to provide evidence in your everyday work that you are able to fulfil all role-specific tasks in accordance with the NMC code and your area's local practice policies.

After achieving this, and when your preceptor and your manager are satisfied, your preceptorship period will be over. This doesn't mean that your colleagues will abandon ship and leave you aboard to care for everyone by yourself. It just means you need less supervision and support in carrying out your daily duties. You can still ask for help anytime you need it, and that advice network should always be there no matter how many years you've been registered. Don't be surprised if soon, more experienced staff turn to you for advice on some recent updates to practice and techniques; preceptorship may end up being a two-way street with you in the teaching role.

However, if at any time you or your colleagues become concerned about your practice, you may be placed back onto temporary preceptorship to help support you in being the best nurse you can be.

My first job was in a respiratory ward. I always wanted to work here throughout my training and, if I am honest, I was overconfident. I thought I knew it all, but preceptorship was the wake-up call and reality check I needed. It helped me realise I needed help, I had questions I needed answers to and I couldn't do it all by myself. My preceptor saw this before I did and encouraged me to open up. Of course, that's not how I saw it at first. I believed they and the other staff were bullying me, pushing me too hard. It was when I sat down and chatted things through with my line manager that it became clear to me I was missing key parts of my job and needed to listen to what my preceptor was telling me to bring that overconfidence down a level so I could perform my job with a clearer mind. It was so good for me, I just wish I had realised earlier.

(NEWLY REGISTERED NURSE JAMES, WHOSE PRECEPTORSHIP PROGRAMME WAS EXTENDED)

WHAT DOES PRECEPTORSHIP NOT INVOLVE?

Preceptorship is a structured period of transition between being the student and becoming the nurse, a process where new registrants will build confidence, hone abilities and continue their journeys in becoming safe and effective practitioners. The preceptorship process is, however, not a period of mentorship, supervision or a process intended to replace mandatory training.

Yes, there are bound to be areas you didn't cover during your degree or skills that you're not familiar with, but your training should have taught you the basics of being a skilled practitioner. Gaining further skills and knowledge is now up to you to facilitate; this is not the role of your preceptor. They may point out areas you can improve on and suggest how you could do this, but ultimately that's your responsibility.

> *There is an onus on the preceptor to help the preceptee, but that must work both ways. We are more like a guide who will show the best routes for how to reach the mountain summit. It's not our responsibility to carry their bags too or pull them up over the final cliff edge. This is their journey to being a good nurse and if they really want that, they have to listen and take it in. I have had new registrants come to me who have only done the basics. No further training, little interest in exploring other skills. The preceptor doesn't exist to fill that gap.*
>
> **(SENIOR NURSE NANCY, PRECEPTOR).**

If you work in an area that requires you to be able to carry out skills you weren't taught at university, then it is your job to complete training so you can carry out these duties in your role.

If you need to be able to insert catheters, set up high-flow oxygen, debride a wound, oscillate someone's chest or even interpret blood results, and you don't know how to, then it is your responsibility to go and learn how to do these things.

Learning does not stop when you graduate from university. As we have discussed before, nursing is a career that requires life-long learning. Some things you will just need to brush up on, other areas will be a whole new world of honing your nursing expertise, all for the benefit of the patient. We are practitioners, we are professionals and we as nurses are experts in our own right, so we should walk the walk as well as we talk the talk.

You can usually book yourself onto training courses through your area's employee online system. Your manager can also help with getting you onto different courses and giving you study time so you can attend. It doesn't always mean that you do this in your own time, but if you want to get some fancy new skills that aren't a complete necessity for your role and are simply nice to have, then you may need to do this in your own time. However, nine times out of 10 your employer will pay for you to attend these courses. If not, check out your union's learning and development section. For instance, the Royal College of Nursing (RCN) has regular courses for nurses of all levels in multiple different areas and is aimed at various specialities. Just check it out.

THE BENEFITS

There are a number of benefits of preceptorship not only for the preceptee but for their employers, their colleagues and patients. Take a look at Table 4.1 highlighting these benefits.

TABLE 4.1 ■ **Benefits of Preceptorship**

Newly Registered Nurse	Preceptor	Employer	Nursing Profession
Helps to build confidence and integration into the new workplace	Assists with appraisals and revalidation	Reduces sickness absence as staff have greater job satisfaction and feel supported	Staff with up-to-date and evidence-based knowledge and practice leading to better patient/client outcomes
Provides support and feedback systems to help encourage reflection in action	Encourages career development and goals for the future	Better outcomes for patients/clients, which improves outlook of the organisation	Enhanced image of the nursing profession and/or that of the organisation
Feels valued as a team member and by their organisation, which leads to job satisfaction and/or improved patient outcomes	Feels valued as an important team member and employee of their organisation, which leads to job satisfaction and/ or improved patient outcomes	Reduced risk of complaints or incidents	Improved public perception and increase in trust in the profession
Allows for structured learning and development	Supports life-long learning and ensures skills and evidence-based practice is up to date	Staff identifying with life-long learning, which enforces change and development	Encourages life-long learning and career development

> *Being able to give feedback to my preceptee made me reflect on my own practice and what areas I could improve in. This made me think more about what I am doing each day and why, meaning my patients are getting the most up-to-date and evidence-based care I can provide – it's a great feeling.*
>
> **(GERRY, A PRECEPTOR OF A NEWLY REGISTERED NURSE)**

CHALLENGES YOU MAY FACE

Despite all of the benefits listed above, you may face challenges during your preceptorship, or even establishing a preceptorship for that matter. Some of these challenges include:

- **Unsafe staffing levels:** Meaning no preceptor available and/or you're expected to work without adequate support in place. If this happens, follow the policy for raising and escalating concerns and discuss it with your line manager (and union if you feel necessary). On this occasion, you will be raising two concerns. One, that you've not had access to a preceptor; and two, unsafe staffing levels (remember, you're accountable, so this is your business and duty under the code).

- **Uninterested preceptor:** This is a tough one, and few people will relish a conversation that more than implies a work colleague is not doing what their role demands. However, remember that besides the patients' needs, this is your career, your life and your mental health. If you have a preceptor who isn't helping you, who is rude or demeaning, or who you know is giving you the wrong guidance, you owe it to yourself to raise that issue with your line manager. In many cases, a quiet word with your preceptor may clear the air of any confusion, but there are occasions when it can go beyond that into bullying or advice which could lead to unsafe practice. By the time you begin your preceptorship, those years of training should begin to hone those nursing instincts about when something is wrong. Use them. Talk to friends or colleagues you trust and seek their advice about whether your concerns are genuine, or if there is a reason why they have been hard or harsh with you. Is there something you need to re-evaluate about your approach to the preceptorship? Or, is your instinct right and they just aren't fulfilling their side of the bargain? If you have concerns, raise them. Ultimately, that's how we best serve the patients, by doing things to the highest standard.
- **Workplace culture:** 'This is how things are done here' – The saying that sends shivers down the spine of any good, self-respecting nurse. If someone says this to you because you challenge what they are teaching, then you know you've got to: first, have evidence to back up your practice; and second, the courage to stand up and say 'well maybe that isn't the way things should be done' … enough said.
- **Bullying and harassment:** We will go into more detail in another chapter, but as a quick point of reference, you are a registered professional. Yes, you are new, but you deserve respect and dignity just like anyone else. Speak up if you're feeling bullied or harassed.

The preceptorship should be an exciting staging post in your development and almost act as a bridge from student to full-fledged nurse. Consider it the final heave into a career which could last decades and take you from adventure to adventure. Relish it, make it exciting and try to avoid seeing it as just another bit of work. It can depend on your preceptor, but take responsibility for what you want to get from it. You might regret not taking full advantage of this time and the opportunities for development it can provide.

To help with this, below are some questions to help focus your mind on what your aims and objectives are for the preceptorship process. Make some bullet points, come back to them a couple of times during your preceptorship, and judge whether you are making the most of it.

Or, if you are currently in the middle of your preceptorship, reflect on what you thought it would be and whether there is time to correct any wrongs or get more from it in the time you have left. We may be graduated professionals by this point, but every day is a school day in nursing.

- **What do I want from my preceptorship?**
  (Ok, so it's that sleepless, restless night before you start your first day. What do you feel most insecure about in your role? What would a guiding hand help you with most?)

  ....
  ....
  ....
  ....
  ....
  ....
  ....
  ....

- **What do I expect it to be like?**
  (Are my expectations for preceptorship realistic? Should I have that conversation before I start with my preceptor about what they will bring to the engagement to figure out what my expectations should be?)

  ....
  ....
  ....
  ....
  ....
  ....
  ....
  ....

■ **How can I make the most of it?**
(Can I be more open about my needs and what I can improve on? How will I ask those questions and seek help?)

....

....

....

....

....

....

....

....

■ **How will I measure my success?**
(Should I write lists or keep a diary? Is there a way of monitoring my progress or seeking feedback every so often to evaluate if I am on the right path?)

....

....

....

....

....

....

....

....

CHAPTER 5

Nursing the Nation

In the darkest hours, the nurse is there. In Bangor, County Down, Northern Ireland, there is a mural depicting a nurse, wearing scrubs, with angel wings behind them. It was a tribute, like many in towns and cities across the United Kingdom, to the health workers who nursed the nation through the COVID-19 pandemic.

The imagery is similar to a well-versed saying we have heard many times as nurses: *'Not all superheroes wear capes.'*

And how true it is.

For months, we wore masks, gloves and visors too. We sanitised, we cleaned, we sprayed and disinfected. In our work we were there for those who needed, despite the intense pressure. We nursed, we cared and we took it home with us, experiencing the same traumatic and life-disturbing events that everyone else was going through.

The spotlight was on nursing like never before, but then that is a light which rarely diminishes.

This is a chapter about how nurses really are superheroes in our own right – and how, like them, we are often called to serve and feel the weight and expectation on our shoulders when the heat is on.

How do we do it? Nurse brain, nurse instinct, that feeling in your gut … this is an attempt to explain it. Nursing is a 24/7 job. Make no mistake about it, you will need those instincts whether you are on shift or not.

Consider the scenario: You come across a road accident before an ambulance has arrived, or you see someone has collapsed in a supermarket. Or – and it doesn't just happen in the films – how would you react if you see someone choking or becoming unwell on a plane?

When the nurse bat signal goes up, the nurse superhero answers.

We are also the dial-a-nurse, an unofficial resource for family and friends, who will call upon you for every ailment. It usually starts with the *'I'm sorry, I know you're not working, but does this rash look weird'* – cue photo being sent to your phone of said rash.

It can sometimes be overwhelming, when all we need after a 12-hour shift is to switch off, that we exist as a reference point for everyone around us.

Of course, this has its benefits. We can spot the signs and intervene to look after those dearest to us. What might have been a long night in an emergency department can be fended off with a triaged phone call.

Always on Call

Here is Aoife, who explains what it can be like to be the *'always nurse-on-call'*:

> *Today, on my day off, I sat in a coffee shop with my laptop and a coffee trying to catch up on some work, but once again found myself 'nursing'. While trying to*

relax after a mental few days on the ward, I heard the high-pitch screaming of a three-month-old boy in the arms of his worn-out-looking mother who was trying her best to pacify him while entertaining her two-year-old girl who was trying to draw on the walls of the newly renovated coffee shop.

I tried not to care, to be selfish and focus on my uncompleted work for my revalidation…but I couldn't. I stood up, smiled at the mum and offered my support. She looked at me as if all her Christmases came at once, and right there I knew where my 'reward' lay.

She was grateful for my non-judgemental and unassuming support unlike the grumpy old man who huffed and puffed as he stormed out of the coffee shop almost blowing it down as he exited.

It is important for nurses to switch off and enjoy the world around us without being on heightened alert. As much as the general public would like to think otherwise, we aren't invincible, we don't have supersoldier strength like Captain America, we are humans, not robots; while what we do for a living is pretty incredible and worthy of superhero status (I may be biased here), in the end we are just normal people who go through the same struggles as everyone else. Burnout is real and can easily slip into our daily lives. But what is the alternative in some situations – do you walk by? Do you pretend you did not see? Do you have a good reason for doing so if you were in a position to help?

We may not know it all or have all the tools at our disposal to help in the moment, but in most situations nurses understand the body and sense the dangers. Part of this comes from that burning desire to help people. It cannot be quantified, but to become a nurse implies you have an innate want to be caring towards others.

Nurse Brain

The other element is experience. With most jobs, procedure becomes instinct. Do something enough times, and practice makes perfect. It is an ability to make a quick assessment and know, without it being easy to explain, exactly the right thing to do at that moment. What am I hearing or seeing, your mind asks. Have I dealt with this before? What did I do?

Imagine how quick you can type on a keyboard or text on your phone. It is instinct, and you might even be able to do it without looking. But have you ever considered how jumbled up the letters would look to someone who has never used a QWERTY keyboard – so named because of how the letters are assembled in the top row?

It might even seem alien that we have this instinct, but through practice our brain processes the information without skipping a beat. And if we mistype a letter, it can be a mild annoyance that we did so.

Fundamentally, the human body has not evolved or changed much in the modern nursing we put into practice today. Some conditions and some bodies are more complex, of course, than others, but we have textbooks about the functions of organs and how our bodies respond when attacked by viruses and disease. We consume that information during our studies to put, as we have discussed in other chapters, our learning into practice.

But some parts of the role are different – they are what we sense as nurses.

As you go through your career, you will come to appreciate the deeper meaning behind the words spoken – and unspoken – in your conversations with patients, their families, maybe even your colleagues. Their tone of voice perhaps belies the words they are using. They say 'I'm OK', but with the inflection in their voice, and the spirit with which they said it, they actually imply they are not. This could also translate into times when someone is in pain.

We have a knack as nurses that by holding the hand of a patient you can tell their response. It can be a great comfort to them, and you sense it in the pressure they use, or do not use.

They act chatty and bubbly one instant, and then you catch them off guard passing by their slightly ajar side room door, and the look in their eyes tell you a different story – the real story.

A truth we must all appreciate is that – one would assume – few people want to require our services. It usually means they, or someone they care about, are unwell – and despite our best efforts to improve their lives, our involvement is by nature a removal of some element of their independence.

They need us, rather than want.

Aoife continued:

I told my husband this story when I got home, and he asked me why I helped this total stranger.

My response was simple: because I'm a nurse.

Nursing for me is about keeping people safe, protecting the vulnerable and caring for those in need. It doesn't matter whether that is in a clinical setting or in the local coffee shop on an ordinary Wednesday afternoon. Nursing isn't always about clinical interventions; sometimes all the person needs is a helping hand or someone to listen. I am a nurse in and out of uniform; I am never really off duty, and I wouldn't have it any other way.

Florence Nightingale – well, of all chapters, this is one she has to be quoted in – once described nursing as an art form.

She operated in an environment far removed from the technology we have today, but she knew there was a craft at the core of being a good nurse.

She also spoke of there being a need for a devotion to the job – a career of passion and preparation.

That to be a good nurse required patience and practice with one's abilities.

Many of us have the caring part but question the skills that make a good nursing instinct.

Are you a problem solver? Could you – and this obviously is not advised in practice – recognise medications by their shape, or know instinctively, as a sixth sense, how much time has passed without looking at a clock?

It is amazing the skills we develop which cannot be judged on a curriculum vitae (CV) but are the little things which accumulate to become integral to what we are as nurses.

Trust Your Instincts

Take a look at Autumn's story below:

I was a newly registered nurse on a busy respiratory ward. On this particular shift, I was nursing a gentleman who was admitted the evening before with multiple rib fractures following an accident. My first interaction with this gentleman was early in the morning before ward round had started. I was checking his observations and administering his regular medications and some pain relief as he complained of pain, which with fractured ribs was to be expected. His blood and observations were all within normal limits and on paper he looked to be doing well. However, my instincts told me otherwise. When I looked at him, his eyes told me something wasn't right. I asked how the patient felt; he explained he was sore and uncomfortable. I tried my best to help ease his pain and discomfort.

The ward round soon began, and I mentioned that I had a gut feeling something else was going on with this patient to one of the senior doctors. This doctor put his hand on my shoulder, looked me in the eyes and told me that I should just listen to him, nothing was wrong, I was overreacting and that I had a lot still to learn but that would come with time. I was shocked and embarrassed, I questioned my own judgement; was I overreacting? Did I get it wrong? I felt stupid, especially as all the other staff including junior doctors and medical students were also on the ward round.

I spent the better half of the morning letting my red face calm down but also taking my time to closely monitor this patient. Despite everything, I felt it in my gut that there was something else going on.

As the day went on, the patient's oxygen requirements increased as his saturations decreased, his pain became worse, he developed what could be described as a chesty cough, and I became more concerned. I escalated this to the medical team. I was told that the patient was fine, and I should just follow the senior doctor's orders from the morning. I was getting nowhere, so I went to the nurse in charge. I explained my concerns, so he came with me to review the patient. Immediately he agreed something wasn't right. He called in the senior doctor who had told me I was overreacting. He reluctantly came to assess the patient. Before I knew it, we were moving the patient's bed, setting up high-flow oxygen and administering intravenous antibiotics. I later heard the nurse in charge speak to the senior doctor about the situation. He told him that, yes, I was a new nurse and I do still have a lot to learn, but this experience shows that so does he.

From that day forward, if I expressed a concern or gut feeling about a patient,
this doctor listened to me and took my opinion on board. It just goes to show that if
your gut and your instinct is telling you there is something wrong, trust them. Ask
advice of other colleagues and always err on the side of caution. It is always better
to ask for help rather than regret keeping quiet.

(AUTUMN, NEWLY REGISTERED NURSE)

What Autumn's story teaches us is that we should always look at the bigger picture. A patient at first glance may appear to be doing well, their blood observations, amongst other investigations, may appear promising, but what else is there for you to explore? How does your patient feel? How do they describe their pain? You know they will be sore – fractured ribs are a nightmare, we know that – but how intense is the pain? Can they describe how it feels? Sharp, dull, piercing? The patient's oxygen saturations are reading normal on the saturation monitor, but does the patient experience any discomfort breathing in or out? How does their chest sound? You don't need to know how to oscillate a chest; you just need to listen to the patient's breathing and identify if something sounds out of place.

It is a puzzle, and you have the job of connecting all the pieces together. If you feel like something just doesn't fit, then speak up. If your gut is telling you something else is happening, then nine times out of 10, it is.

I once worked with a senior doctor who was very skilled and great at his job. Even if he had just assessed a patient and found no new issues, if one of the nurses went to him and said, *'So doctor, I have this feeling that* [insert your concern here],' he always trusted us, and used to say jokingly, *'You nurses, your instincts and gut feelings are making me earn my salary today.'*

Perhaps the moral of the story is: trust your gut, even if you feel like you're overreacting. Always air on the side of caution and reach out for help. This is not a drill or a trial run; you have real peoples' lives in your hands, so if you feel something isn't right, explore that feeling and ask for help.

Autopilot

When something's happening, you go on autopilot, and adrenaline carries you through. Have you ever felt like you are just coasting through life: you've dropped the kids off to school, took the dog for a walk, made coffee and now you're sitting at your desk in work wondering, how? How did I do all of that before 9 am? Did I remember to lock the front door?

Have you driven to work and got to the car park and thought to yourself, *'I don't even remember how I got here'*?

Everyone experiences autopilot in their daily lives. You know how to make a cup of coffee without thinking. You brush your teeth without even considering what you're doing. As humans, we have an incredible ability to retain memory. From our first breaths our bodies learn how to breathe without it being a conscious act. Many of our nursing abilities come naturally too.

How many times recently have you thought about how to apply a blood pressure cuff to obtain a blood pressure reading? Have you really thought about the steps you take when you are obtaining blood, drawing up a medication or emptying a catheter? No? Do you do this in autopilot? Do these tasks soon become second nature?

Take this, for example: You're out shopping with a friend who suddenly takes ill, complaining of feeling light-headed and dizzy. Without a second thought, your first action is to identify several possibilities in a mental checklist. First, what are the symptoms – headache, feeling weak and clammy. Next is the sub-symptoms: they don't have any pain but how do they feel? You tick each off as you rattle through them. You soon realise that your friend has skipped lunch and needs food. Your next stop on your shopping day is a cafe for some lunch and thankfully not the local emergency department after your friend collapses.

Another example is choking. You're in a restaurant having dinner. You hear the sounds of a young girl coughing. Her family doesn't seem alarmed at first, but you hear the cough differently and identify it as choking. The parents can't hear this, they're offering water, but you've already set a countdown timer in your mind. You know you need to act, so you do. Soon you're at their table administering back slaps, and eventually a large piece of steak is dislodged and the girl begins to get her colour back.

What if your mum tells you she just doesn't feel right? You know she has type two diabetes and you know she isn't very well controlled. You begin to ask questions, *What did you have to eat today?'* … *'Have you checked your sugars recently, what were they?'* … *'Have you had all of your medications this morning?'* Soon you discover your mum has eaten a full bar of chocolate and washed it down with a full-fat soda, and there you have your diagnosis.

In both your personal and nursing life, autopilot plays a major role in helping you get through your days. You arrive at a patient's house for their leg ulcer wound dressing change. You go to your boot and lift out everything you need to complete this task. You change the dressing while talking to your patient about knitting patterns and the weather. Yes, you are focused on the task at hand but you are able to do this instinctively while conducting a conversation with this patient.

But what if next time you visit this patient's house you see a sink full of dishes, expired milk in the fridge and the patient appears unkempt. The patient is smiling, delighted to see you; after all you are the only visitor they have. You think about this patient on your journey home, before you switch off your bedroom lamp and when you wake in the morning.

Unfortunately some people experience devastating traumas in their lives, some unthinkable experiences which have resulted in them being in your care. You're the person there to help pick up the pieces and mend parts of their lives. You go through this with them and, yes, that can be a pleasure, but it can also be completely devastating for you too.

If you begin to take work home, think about your patients on your days off and feel like you've nothing left to give, remember why you started.

Like the boxer who has a title to win but keeps getting knocked to the canvas, just like they find the strength to rise to their feet, nurses should support each other to get back up as well.

However, if you ever get to a stage where you simply cannot go on, you feel overwhelmed, stressed and ready to give up, then it may be time to admit you are experiencing burnout.

Emotional Challenges

In this line of work, it is no shock that you will experience emotional challenges, some of patients and their experiences, but mostly you will have experiences that will affect you personally.

Some experiences will affect you in the moment, others you will take home to digest. Then there are other incidents that you just can't get out of your head. You relive that moment every time you walk into the room it happened, every time you carry out similar tasks or hear of the same diagnosis. This is when you need to take the gloves off and step out of the ring. This is when you need to realise you are burnt out.

Stress and Burnout

Enter burnout – the state of both physical and emotional exhaustion.

It is almost a guarantee that you will feel stress and potentially burnout during your nursing life. Faced with some of the situations we encounter, you would be right to question: How can you avoid them?

However, here is another healthy reminder to plead with you to seek support. Stress has never been solved by bottling it away, pretending it does not exist. Instead, it can fester and pester, growing to cause real lasting harm.

Instead, be open about your feelings. You will be surprised at the level of stress being experienced by others around you also, even if they do not show it. You are not alone and there is help available.

Here are some signs to watch out for, and know to admit, when you are feeling close to breaking point.

The National Health Service (NHS) lists them as follows:

- Feeling overwhelmed
- Experiencing racing thoughts or difficulty concentrating
- Becoming irritable
- Feeling worried, anxious or scared
- Lacking self-confidence
- Trouble sleeping or feeling tired all the time
- Avoiding things or people you associate problems with
- Eating, drinking or smoking more or less than usual

Your friends and family may point out your stress triggers, things which cause you to become anxious or timid, annoyed or strained. Many people like to go through life as if their problems are not worthy of attention, but try to judge whether speaking out could help.

Alongside professional help and advice, trying to manage your downtime to do things you enjoy may help. A more fixed sleeping pattern may help too. Reading more, exercise, learning a new craft – there are many resources out there which can provide tips about ways to reduce stress. It is, however, easier said than done when we work in such a pressured environment.

Remember, you are not a superhero with invincible powers like in the movies. As much as we don't want to admit it, we nurses are human too. The public may have this perception of us as angels, heroes and resilient, and we are all of those things, but we can't be them all the time. We aren't robots, we are humans, just like anyone else. When our tank is empty, we too need to be refuelled. Sometimes, this refuelling may come in the form of time off from work and speaking to our occupational health department or our managers. If you need help, please ask for it. As the saying goes, you can't help others if you are burning your candle at both ends.

If you feel stressed or burnt out:

- Speak with your colleagues – you may just need some support on those extra tough days.
- Have a conversation with your manager – they may be able to help shield you from intense areas for a little while so you can have some breathing space.
- Talk to your loved ones – we know we can't divulge patient details to our families, but you do need to talk. Explain your feelings and how they are affecting you, but in a way that protects the patient and their confidentiality.
- Seek counselling – sometimes things just get too much. Have a chat with your doctor, ask for a referral to a counsellor or approach the occupational health department in your work and see what they can offer you.

Bullying and Harassment

Linda is a band 6 specialist nurse with many years of experience and a high skill set. Linda has been working in her current job for around three years and loves it. Her team has recently had a new manager take over who has transferred from another department.

Almost immediately Linda feels like this manager doesn't like her and isn't happy with how she conducts her workload. For example, the new manager is constantly asking Linda to provide her with a breakdown of what she is doing every minute of every day she works. This manager has not requested this from other employees and provides no justification for this request.

The manager asks to see Linda for an update on her caseload. From the outset the manager tells Linda she should do things differently and should rearrange how she conducts her work week.

Linda works part-time hours and has flexible working in place due to caring commitments outside of work. The new manager has told her that she needs to change her hours of work and that she can no longer have set working days, suggesting that Linda needs to be more flexible.

Linda was in the office one morning, with members of the administration team present, and Linda's manager out of the blue asked if she has been looking for other jobs. Linda responded that she hasn't. Her manager simply grunted and continued with her work.

Linda is left feeling humiliated, offended and quite frankly intimidated by this new manager.

List three ways below how you think Linda is being bullied or harassed:

1.

2.

3.

What would you do if you were in Linda's situation?

_____

_____

_____

Bullying and harassment are never acceptable. Whether it is the classroom, the home, the workplace, among friends or colleagues – it is demeaning, cruel, discriminatory and intolerable. We discuss whistleblowing and referring concerns elsewhere in this book, but here it should be stressed that if you are a witness of bullying, it needs to be called out.

The impact it can have on someone's mental health, let alone their ability to practice safely as a nurse, is worthy of your attention. Employers too need to ensure their policies are up-to-date and, following any cases of bullying or harassment, are re-investigated and updated.

Each workplace has a duty of care to its employees. Managers, good ones, look out for their staff and have their back.

Bullying and harassment can of course come in multiple forms: a quick remark, a supposedly funny quip, an unwanted sharing of a meme or a joke. It may seem small and trivial to the sender. It could be an invasion of privacy and deeply offensive to the receiver. Physical and emotional abuse can take its toll. One incident can lead to more. A sustained period of this can cause untold damage, but even that initial incident could be enough to send someone's well-being down a path they do not deserve.

It goes without saying that how we all combat this is to show respect to our colleagues, appreciating the diversity and talents of our teams, promoting inclusivity, calling out those who undermine such efforts and dealing promptly with those who go too far.

For managers, be self-critical. Am I too harsh with them? Do I demand too much? Do they need training rather than me shouting at them for something they cannot yet do?

Most of us will witness, or experience, some form of bullying and harassment. One would hope the perpetrator would realise and apologise for their actions to avoid repetition, depending on the offence. Some things are, however, unforgivable in a workplace. Racism, sexism, sectarianism, misogyny – there is a long list of the unforgivable in the eyes of this author and in the code of the Nursing and Midwifery Council (NMC).

Discrimination can come in many forms. It may not always be direct, sometimes it can be those little comments which bear a weight that at the time may seem insignificant, but on reflection are actually quite a blow to the chest.

Take Oscar's experience, for example, which could involve casual discrimination:

Oscar is a nurse in Northern Ireland where community tensions remain as a legacy of The Troubles. Many decades of bloodshed have created divisions between Protestants and Catholics, those who campaign for a United Kingdom and those who want a united Ireland.

Oscar is at work one afternoon and on the radio he hears a story about trouble involving the bus service he needs to use to get home. Young people have been hijacking buses and setting them alight. Oscar is concerned about how he will get home and asks his manager if he can head home early to avoid any further escalation of the violence.

His manager agrees … but this is how they respond, making Oscar reflect on the situation during his journey home.

> **Manager:** *'Yes Oscar, head on home. Sure when you get to where the trouble is you jump off and join in, sure it's your side causing all this anyway.'*
>
> **Oscar:** *'What do you mean my side?'*
>
> **Manager:** *'Oh, I'm just joking. Have a safe trip home. Let me know you get to your house okay.'*

Oscar is already worried about his journey, and now he has been left to ponder what his manager meant. Was he being deliberately or accidentally sectarian? Did he really think he was the type to get involved in something so destructive? Would he have said this if he had known he was, in fact, from a different part of the community than those committing the trouble, which is why he was in such fear? The next day, Oscar does his best to avoid the subject with his manager, concerned about where the conversation could lead.

How do you feel after reading Oscar's interaction with his manager? Do you feel this was sectarian? Is he making too much out of it to be concerned?

Was the manager out of line? Could it damage his trust with his manager in the future?

Where Can You Get Support?

If you feel you are experiencing bullying or harassment, you need to speak up and get help. The impact bullying and harassment can have is frightening; we need to know there is help and support out there for all of us.

Nurses talk about emotional well-being and being mindful – we need to put this advice into practice and help ourselves. Sometimes the approach can be simple; it may just result in a conversation with the aggressor. Other times it will be more complex, and we may have some trauma from the incidents which will require further support and help. This is where it is essential to know where to turn.

In some instances, it can be difficult to seek help. You may feel worried that by reporting this behaviour and accessing support it could cause further problems, but if you don't speak up, then things will continue to spiral. Would you walk past bad care? Would you keep quiet if you witnessed a patient being bullied or harassed? What would you do if you realised a patient was experiencing racial, physical or emotional abuse? Would you keep quiet?

I hope your answer for all of those questions is a resounding no.

So if you would stand up, speak up and be an advocate for your patients, why wouldn't you do the same for yourself or your colleagues?

Whistleblowing on bullying or harassment can be scary and worrying, but what is the outcome if you don't act? Do you leave a job you love? Do you take your feelings and anger towards the situation home to your family?

Michelle Obama once said, 'When they go low, we go high'.

So rise above the person or the people who are bullying and harassing you. You are better than them to sink to their level by inflicting the same behaviour on someone else. You haven't done anything wrong and, as the say, karma will follow: what goes around comes around.

Here are some tips on dealing with bullying and harassment:

- **Speak to a manager:** In the first instance speak to your line manager. Ask to do so confidentially and discuss an action plan for the next steps. Naturally if the line manager is the person causing you problems, you may need to turn to another senior colleague for guidance.
- **Ask your union for help:** If you want help but you feel as though you need support or guidance around your employer's policies on resolving such matters, then always contact your trade union for information. They may be able to represent you, or sit in on meetings with management. You pay your union fees for such help, so do not be afraid to ask for it.
- **Keep a diary of events:** It can be really important during the investigation process that there is documented evidence of bullying or harassment incidents. Even if this is your own thoughts and feelings on the incident, writing this down at the time and marking the date/time can be crucial. If you don't feel comfortable writing this in a notebook, then email yourself. Write down the contents of the incident at the time or as close to the time of incident as possible. Email this account to a personal email address and keep a diary this way. This will be date and time stamped and provide you with a method of building a portfolio of evidence over the course of however long this bullying or harassment lasts. You can print and use these emails as your evidence of events.
- **Speak to someone you trust:** Even if this person is a family member or a close friend, get your feelings off your chest and talk them through with someone.

Don't bottle up how you feel. What would you say to a patient if they were in the same boat?

- **Check your employer's local policy:** Each workplace should have a policy on how to deal with bullying and harassment claims, including informal and formal actions. Your employer has a legal responsibility and duty of care for the health and safety of its employees under the Health and Safety at Work Act 1974, the Equality Act 2010 and the Protection from Harassment Act 1997. Each employer should encourage staff to report incidents of bullying or harassment and, where appropriate, take disciplinary actions towards the aggressor while supporting and protecting the victim of this behaviour.

But what if you are being bullied by a patient or their family member?

Any type of bullying or harassment is difficult and can be challenging to deal with, but it can be even more testing when the aggressor is a patient in your care or their family members.

Let's take a look at Leanne's story.

'Today I was nursing a patient, a gentleman, let's call him Barney. Barney reported to me that the toilet in the en-suite of his side room wasn't flushing properly. I reported the problem to our estates team who came immediately to resolve the issue. The estates team informed me they could fix the problem but would need to replace the toilet. They could do this right away. I informed Barney who at this point was ambulating around the ward as advised by his surgical team. Barney seemed happy that the problem was being sorted. I told him he could use our television room during the repair and if he needed anything to let me know; we unfortunately didn't have any spare beds to move him to. Soon it was visiting time. Barney's wife appeared on the ward along with his sister. I walked to them to explain that Barney was in the television room enjoying a cup of tea and some football and informed them of the ongoing repairs in Barney's room.

Barney's family didn't seem pleased and walked passed me to their loved one. A little time passed. I was in the clinical room drawing up some medications when I heard a commotion from the nurses' station. I popped my head out to see what was going on. I overheard Barney's wife shouting at a colleague, stating: 'He has had surgery and he is in a room where a toilet is being replaced, all the infection is now in the air, what if it goes into his wound, he should be in his bed, not sitting on a chair'.

My colleague tried to reassure his wife, but she kept shouting louder. I locked my medications away and approached Barney's wife; after all, I was his nurse. I introduced myself again to her and asked how I could help. What followed was loud shouting, threats against me and a lot of choice words. I let Barney's wife speak. When I felt the time was right, I asked her to let me speak. I asked if she would mind lowering her tone and if she would refrain from using derogatory and threatening language towards me. I made Barney's wife aware of the zero tolerance of abuse of staff policy and asked if she could take some time to cool down.

We could then speak after. I asked her to either leave the ward or go back to her husband and I would speak to her soon.

During this time I looked up and printed out our complaints procedure; I also printed out the zero tolerance policy and made our nurse in charge aware of the situation. I also asked one of our healthcare assistants to come with me as a witness during my next interactions.

I approached the television room and made sure it was only Barney and his family present. I closed the door and asked if we could speak. I introduced my colleague and asked Barney if he would like to raise a concern regarding the situation. Barney declined and said he was happy watching his favourite football team beat their rivals. I asked Barney's wife how she felt; she was still angry and proceeded to shout at me and criticise my abilities as a nurse.

I asked her to calm down and warned her that if she continued, I would have her removed from the ward. This only angered her further. I informed her that her husband's room was ready for use, it had been cleaned following the toilet repair, and there were no further issues identified. I also informed her that we have a zero-tolerance policy for abuse towards staff, and if she would like to raise a concern or complaint, we were happy to assist in any possible way. I left the complaints procedure and the zero-tolerance policies with her. I left the room and informed her the nurse in charge would be in touch.

Some time later the nurse in charge informed me that Barney's wife had declined proceeding with a complaint and had apologised for her behaviour. She had since left the ward. Barney's team won the match and he was tucked up in bed with a cup of tea. Nothing more was said on the matter.'

Did Leanne handle the situation well?

_____

_____

_____

List two things you would have done in this situation:

1. _____

_____

_____

2. _____

_____

_____

It can be difficult to approach any situation where you feel like you are being bullied or harassed. Leanne's story shows us how this can happen so easily, and unfortunately in some instances nurses can feel threatened that they may even be assaulted for doing their job. It doesn't always have to be a colleague or a manager who inflicts work-related bullying or harassment. It is therefore fundamental you are aware of your workplace's local policies on such behaviour. Look these up and familiarise yourself with their contents so if you are ever in a situation like Leanne, you will know how to act.

Our job is hard enough as it is. Dealing with bullying and harassment could happen during your career; hopefully not, but it is something we must always be alert to so it can be ended at the earliest opportunity.

I hope this chapter has provided some hints and tips for how to deal with such situations. The key takeaway from this chapter is that you are not alone and there is support out there if you ever need it.

CHAPTER 6

Putting Your Research and Evidence Into Practice

Nursing has a proud history, with the modern profession built on the practices and principles that have been passed from one generation of carers to the next.

So, when you hear the term 'evidence-based practice', do not fear the academic undertone of this, but embrace the fact that what you should do as a nurse will be backed up by well-trodden ideas that have been shown to be effective.

In daily life, when you have an experience, it should influence your future actions. Consider it to be a form of self-research, whereby if something goes wrong, you should try to learn a lesson or seek ways to eliminate mistakes in future. By doing so, you reduce risk and find methods that will make your life easier and your prospects more successful. Well, that's the hope anyway.

The purpose of research follows a similar path. Find a problem, test a theory, put the research into practice, judge if it works or not. Then, if it does, roll it out as wide as possible. We have seen this with many studies. Think about the COVID-19 vaccine and treatments that emerged within mere months into the pandemic. Researchers worked frantically to test ways to combat the virus and expose their data to reviews, and what happened afterwards made history, as both vaccines and antiviral drugs soon emerged, which changed the lives of millions.

In your career, whether indeed you become a research nurse or any of the other lines of work we examined in Chapter two, you should try to cling onto that inner student; the one you hoped you left behind with your final exams.

Yes, those painful late nights studying will be replaced by long days of work, but the danger for any medical professional is to slip into the 'I know it all' mindset.

Nurses are carers but also problem solvers. Hand us a complex issue with a patient, and like any health professional, we try to diagnose and find solutions for them as best as we can. The nurse's brain and instinct can only take you so far. Everything else is based on a basic level of study and the training and research we consume thereafter to inform our next actions.

Many patients would not have survived without nurses keeping an inquisitive mind to put emerging research into practice. As we have previously pondered, the nurses who tended to soldiers in field hospitals at war, or, for instance, those who nursed bomb and gun attack victims during the Northern Ireland Troubles, have taken what was known before and built on it for their own circumstances. Their actions led to research. We now put the evidence from that research into practice.

You can be the best nurse in your field, outstanding in your knowledge of medicines and techniques. You may have skills in dealing with patients undergoing mental trauma or an ability to speak to someone about a dying relative. However, sometimes we need to admit we do not know everything—or, take a moment to question if we can do things better.

Do not let your busy life at work distract you from seeking out the wealth of research and information that emerges each year, challenging some long-held beliefs and bringing forward ideas that, if applied, could save you time and resources, perhaps even lives. Research does not just benefit specialists; it is available and useful to all.

Keep in mind that research underpins our accountability. We are all judged by standards, much of which will have been directly or indirectly based on previous research. The Nursing and Midwifery Council (NMC) Code has ultimately developed from prior studies—that is how the NMC knows the code works. When methods are shown to be effective, they become part of our practice. If we deviate from or fall short of those standards, it is against the code and against those rules where nurses can be found accountable. Hence the importance of training and consuming research. Keep yourself up to speed with what is expected from a modern nurse and you should be an effective practitioner.

Think of the patient. Or, rather, imagine you are the patient. If your nurse explains that they are trying out a new type of injection on your arm or a new technique for taking blood, you would want to know that it has been well tested before it comes anywhere near you. It will certainly breed more confidence than learning you were a test case for something which had not been well researched.

In a court environment, judges will listen to cases and base their decisions on the law of the land as well as how previous similar cases have laid down precedents for what they should do. In the same way, a nurse should use evidence-based research. A judge cannot make a ruling on a whim. They have to know they can back it up and point to why they ruled the way they did.

In this chapter, we will explore the different types of research, how to use them and why they help. We will also provide examples of how research and evidence underpin and shape our practice daily.

As we go, ask yourself if you could do more to research areas of your work or if there are studies you have found interesting which would be worth sharing with colleagues.

What Is the Difference Between Quantitative and Qualitative Research?

There are many types of research, but let's focus initially on the two forms which are most well known, quantitative and qualitative, and how they differ.

I know what you're thinking: *'Why do I need to know the different types of research when I am just starting out?'* Well, it is simple. If you want to ensure your practice is always backed by evidence and how this works in reality, then knowing the difference between the most well-known types of research can give you a head start in finding research to support you and your actions.

I know understanding research can be difficult for some. I too struggled to understand the basics of research during my degree. It was one of the modules at the university I dreaded; I know I am not alone in that.

But (there's always a but), all those years later, here I am now, writing this chapter having worked as a research nurse, and I can tell you it is actually a lot more straightforward than it may appear at first.

I have had first-hand experience of how research has both informed and improved my practice, and I have seen how research has transformed care. More on that later, but for now, let's tackle the two Qs, as I like to call them: quantitative and qualitative research.

Quantitative Research

When you hear quantitative, think quantity. Something you can measure based on an amount. This tends to be data and numbers driven, with clear figures used to assess a result. For instance, if an action occurs X number of times, what impact does it have on a patient's heart rate or blood pressure? This form of research can be simpler to measure and lends itself to being presented with clear charts and graphs to show trends.

The challenge for the author or conductor of this type of research is to present their findings as well as their methods in a clear way. Can their study be replicated with the same results if reviewed by their peers?

Are there any elements of the research which would not hold up to scrutiny and have influenced the study?

Okay, now let us look at this using something we should all know about: National Early Warning Scores, or NEWS. So most of us have used the NEWS system at some stage. Maybe you use it regularly if you are a ward nurse, or perhaps you just remember it from placements. Regardless of your experience, I am sure we can all agree that it is a pretty great system that helps indicate our patient's condition.

NEWS is a system which allows us as practitioners to visually see how good or bad our patient's vital signs are by using numbers and colours. Using a traffic light system, NEWS allows us to track patients' blood pressure, heart rate, oxygen saturations, temperature, respiration rates and even their blood sugar levels (NEWS may differ throughout the United Kingdom—I am basing this on my experience in Northern Ireland). At the end, we have a number score which indicates good, not so good and… yeah… we need to worry. It is simple—the higher the number, the sicker the patient.

But how do we know that this system works? Did someone, one day, just decide they wanted to add a little colour to observation charts and a fun adding game? No… this system was tried and tested before it was rolled out across healthcare and the UK. Its success speaks for itself.

BOX 6.1 ■ Example

Consider this: you work in a busy surgical ward with a high rate of patients who deteriorate after surgery. You want to investigate why this happens and examine if there are any developing trends. So, you take a look at the observation charts of patients who have deteriorated after surgery.

You collect the data about their observations post-surgery until they deteriorated. You notice that in five out of six patients, the systolic blood pressure is low. The blood pressure of these patients jumps up and down, ranging from 70 to 90 systolic. You then start to notice

Continued

BOX 6.1 ■ **Example**—cont'd

the heart rates of these patients beginning to climb. Next, we have lower oxygen saturations, forcing higher levels of oxygen therapy. In all, a classic cycle of the deteriorating patient.

You then compare these findings with patients who did not experience a deterioration after surgery. You notice these patients have blood pressures ranging from 100 systolic and greater. You dig deeper and find these patients had intravenous fluids on their return to the ward.

Is there a trend here? Have the intravenous fluids prevented deterioration? As a result of your findings, your ward develops a policy that it is mandatory that all patients returning after surgery to be assessed and considered for maintenance intravenous fluids in order to prevent hypotension leading to deterioration.

The research you carried out to assess how intravenous fluids prevented higher levels of hypotension and thus forward patient decline used quantitative methods as it involved measuring numbers.

You may already be carrying out research by assessing your patients without even knowing it.

Qualitative Research

This is much harder to measure and can focus more on feelings, as opposed to something with identifiable numbers. If an action happens, how does the patient respond? If they are undergoing a certain type of procedure, how do they feel?

This type of research can have its detractors who point to the individualised experience, which is very difficult to replicate with other studies.

It will need to be based on information gathered genuinely from the participants of the study, but can the variety of responses be useful?

In many ways, this type of research can lead to further theories which can be tested, or a deeper analysis can be made to see how experiences change over time. The results can be extremely useful to assess how patients may feel when something happens. By examining this, we can find ways to better handle situations, such as breaking bad news or how to help a patient's recovery based on how others have responded.

BOX 6.2 ■ **Example**

You have a group of patients with communication difficulties, a young child or even a patient who does not speak your language. You ask them about their pain, but they find it difficult to convey how they feel. What do you do? You need to know the pain scores of these patients to ensure they are receiving adequate pain relief or consider if they may be receiving pain medication that they do not actually need.

You try asking the question, '*how is your pain?*' in multiple different ways with no result. So, you decide to draw some faces ranging from happy to sad. You ask the patient to point to the face that they are feeling. If they point to the sad face, you know they need more pain relief, and if they point to the happy face, you know they do not.

This method does not use fancy graphs or number scoring. It is not based on data you can see and analyse, but rather it is based on how the patient feels. This is still useful and important data to capture, as it gives you an insight into the condition of a patient who cannot communicate their feelings in the usual way.

HOW IS RESEARCH CONDUCTED?

You will find research under many different guises: from a scholarly article about a specific technique to a root-and-branch review of the wider health system. There is a lot of information out there to peruse.

Let's focus on a couple of areas where you will find most of your information.

CONTROL AND COHORT STUDIES

One of the most common forms of medical research involves a controlled study. This will often require the recruitment of patients with a pre-known condition into a study where, for instance, they are provided with a new drug which is hoped to potentially aid their treatment.

Over time, they will be assessed to see if there has been an improvement. Some studies will introduce a randomised element where some patients are provided with a placebo, or no treatment, to see if there is a different set of results compared to the other patients.

Cohort studies will look at broader sections of the population to see if specified trends are having an impact over time.

When the study has run its course, these findings can be peer-reviewed and could lead to the adoption of new medications for relevant nurses to administer.

BOX 6.3 ■ Example

A doctor specialising in diabetes started prescribing a new drug, let's call it 'sugar low', for his patients with type two diabetes mellitus. He knew this drug had been praised for its ability to lower the HbA1c (blood sugar level) of patients with type two diabetes, and the research even suggested it had also been useful in helping these patients to lose unwanted weight.

However, this doctor soon noticed another trend. Since beginning this drug, his patients who normally suffered from hypertension were experiencing lower blood pressure readings. As a result, this doctor discussed the benefits of sugar low with his cardiologist friend. Together they developed a study which trialed sugar low versus a placebo in patients with type two diabetes to see if the lower blood pressures were in fact as a result of the drug or not.

The findings showed that sugar low was a great drug for lowering blood pressure, controlling type two diabetes and also helping people to lose unwanted weight. In all, a wonder drug. Now, sugar low is used in multiple different settings for patients with different conditions.

SYSTEMIC REVIEW

This type of review is very broad and consists of an examination of all relevant studies about a topic. Generally, this can monitor trends and differences between research projects. The end result can be an overarching picture of whether the results match up and should be adopted.

This can be a time-consuming process, but one that could provide a more forensic appraisal of whether the results should be enacted for patients' benefits.

A meta-analysis is similar to a systematic review, where the statistics from quantitative research projects are combined to give a full set of results and conclusions.

CAN YOU TRUST THE RESEARCH?

As with any source of information, think about who it has been authored by or the publisher. Is it a serious review of data, conducted by a reputable organisation or individual, or do you have doubts about whether the information is true? If you believe in the latter, chances are this is not the type of research you should go near in terms of adopting it into practice as a nurse.

It is our job to be sure of our evidence-based practice. If we question its validity, then either it is unlikely to be trustworthy or it is an area which demands further research before its findings should influence our treatment of patients.

Think back to your essays at university where you searched for research to back up your points. You were advised by your lecturers not to use something you found on 'Dr Google' but to use a source which was well accredited and up to date. Why would you use anything less now? Especially as now you're really using this knowledge to support real-life patients, not those fictionalised in your assignments. The marks here are given by the patient, not your lecturers.

Consider the motivation for the research. Is it testing a hypothesis or a problem you believe exists and where care can be improved? If so, examining the results could be of real benefit, and you may already have an interest in how it can be put into practice.

Has the research been conducted by an academic institution? Or has it been approved by a pharmaceutical company or another firm with a vested interest in how the results should be presented because it wants to influence policy for its benefit? This is not to dismiss research carried out by private enterprises; they can have their uses, but always question the who and the why behind research.

Also keep in mind whether the research has been conducted ethically. Did the participants know fully what they had consented to? Were they misled or were their confidences breached? Have illicit methods been used to find out information? Has the study stated how it carried out the research?

Every research study today must have ethical approval. It is key to making sure the research carried out is done in a manner that protects the participants, the researchers and anyone who may be beneficiaries of the research.

Let's talk about why ethics is important.

When I took up a post as a research nurse, I had to fight my way through a minefield of jargon (no, it doesn't stop when you leave the wards—it actually gets worse) and try to understand why each aspect of approval for a study to commence was so important. I was discussing ethical approval with my manager one afternoon, and she directed me to a report about a research study that was carried out on a group of African American males with syphilis.

This study is known as the *'Tuskegee Syphilis Study'*.

In brief, this study was set up to examine how syphilis would affect the human body if left untreated. However, what makes this study completely unethical is the fact that, by the end of the study, there was a treatment for this disease. However, the participants included in the study were not made aware of this, and more than 100 died as a result.

Protections today are now in place to prevent such failings from occurring again. If a cure or treatment becomes available for a condition or disease, it is up to the study team to be open and honest with participants about this, regardless of what this means for retention or recruitment.

Each presentation of findings should carry a conclusion or an executive summary. This will be the author's final call on how the data and the study should be presented. What they believe are the most important points and, perhaps, what they would like to see happen based on their research. That could be anything from a simple change in methods, which can be quickly adopted, to something which calls into question a strategic policy of the health and care system which will take time and money to implement.

Judge these conclusions by the title or stated aims of the research. Did the research achieve what it set out to? Was the grand question on the title page answered, or did the end findings merely scratch the surface and struggle to get to the heart of the issue? If this is the case, perhaps it was not worth the investment, either by the sponsor or in your time reading it.

Such research, however, can prove to be a staging post for someone else to take on further.

In many ways, all knowledge is useful, whether it answers the question or not. This does not, however, mean we can rely on it for evidence-based practice; quite the opposite.

HOW SHOULD I USE RESEARCH IN PRACTICE?

It is one thing to know the theory, or read the research, but how should you use it in practice?

Well, you started doing this from your first days on placement. It is unlikely that when you first left the confines of the lecture theatre and entered a real nursing environment that your actions were carried out 'on a hunch'. You will have sought advice and help, and used what you learned in the degree to make sure you could back up your decisions on your placement.

As this book has repeated, if you are unsure about something you have experienced, always ask for guidance or support. Few things will ever be worth risking your PIN over. With the help of colleagues, some gaps in knowledge can be easily filled. Generally, with life inside and outside of work, if you receive help, you should question what you didn't know and make sure that if the situation arises again, you are prepared to meet it on your own.

Our end goal is to help patients. New methods based on research should not scare us, but actually be a good thing, as they may make our lives easier too.

You should accept that as you go through your nursing journey, there will be plenty of 'uh-oh' moments. Those little seconds when time freezes, your stomach seizes and you fear you've made a mistake akin to pressing the nuclear button by accident.

Base your work on researched methods, and it should be clearer to anyone you call upon for help what it was you did and how to fix it. Mistakes can happen, and so too can doubts. You may encounter colleagues who subtly suggest, *'I'm not sure that's right'* when they witness your practice. This is a job with high stakes, and we will have times where we doubt if what we did was right. The best way to combat that and to defend our actions is to use evidence-based practice.

In the sense that no two patients are the same, equally, you are not the same as another nurse. We all have different skills and ways of approaching conversations with patients about the care they need.

Nurses need to be critical thinkers and always be inquisitive. That is how we get to the bottom of an ailment suffered by a patient who is perhaps not telling everything about their condition or the circumstances around what happened to them.

As we discuss later in the book, reflection is an important part of our practice as nurses, where we assess our development and seek to learn lessons. As part of reflection, remind yourself of the value of research and how it can feed into your work.

WORK AS A RESEARCH NURSE

As a nurse, you do not just have to use evidence-based practice; you could be part of its formation by becoming a research nurse. Generally, this will require some prior work before you are at a level to apply for such a role, but consider whether it is something that would interest you.

For instance, as a research nurse on a vaccine trial, you could be responsible for follow-up blood tests and conversations with study participants, recording data based on their stats and responses, which will feed into the wider study and later develop treatments or methods which help to stabilise and treat certain conditions and/or diseases.

Or, if a new drug emerges which could help some cancer patients or people who have diabetes, you could be at the forefront of the efforts to improve the lives of millions. The impact of research could help patients both at home and around the world.

Being part of such research could be a badge of honour and bring immense job satisfaction.

Being a research nurse isn't all paperwork and being stuck behind a computer screen or with your nose in books. The role of a research nurse is so versatile. For example, during my first few months working as a research nurse, I covered multiple specialities, including assisting the stroke team on some of their studies.

Being a stroke research nurse means carrying the emergency bleep. So, when a patient is being transferred or admitted to the hospital with a queried stroke, or an inpatient suffers stroke-like symptoms, the bleep goes off and the specialist stroke team all race to these patients. So does the stroke research nurse. You are there on the front line in the emergency department, the hospital ward or the waiting room, assisting in this patient's life-saving care, and on occasion helping the team to distinguish if this patient is suitable for a certain new treatment or not, which may increase their chances of recovery or survival.

These calls definitely get the adrenaline pumping.

Working as a research nurse requires great time management and organisation skills, but it also requires the ability to be a holistic and independent practitioner. Most of the time, it's you who keeps the study running, and without that work, new treatments or methods may not make it across your department's doors.

Conclusions

Good job if you have made it to the end of this chapter. I know some of you would have seen the title and thought, *'yeah, maybe I'll skip that one'*. I, too, would have been guilty of those thoughts in the past.

However, since registering, I now realise why my lecturers at university always drummed on about the importance of evidence-based practice, and why we needed to study research methods.

It's simple: without research we wouldn't have evidence-based practice, and without evidence-based practice we would not be as advanced in health and social care as we are today.

Now that we have covered research and evidence-based practice, let's take a look at reflection and what all the fuss is about.

CHAPTER 7

Reflection: What's All the Fuss About?

Before we discuss why you need to reflect, let's first analyse why you would want to.

Nursing is a fast-paced role. Some of our duties remain the same day-in-day-out, but there are also many variables, and countless opportunities to learn.

The best way to think about reflection is a nursing 'dear diary', a personal account to recall your experiences, both the good and the not-so-good.

You should 'want' to reflect because it is an acknowledgement of your willingness to learn from your mistakes, those little elements of bad practice which can creep in, those lessons from others or words of advice.

It is a self-critical look at where you have room to grow.

The purpose of reflection is about learning, not to only show off your successes or depressingly analyse the lows.

In this book, we use the 'dear diary' analogy because many people will have kept diaries, or notes, at some stage of their life. At the time when they were written, you were at the peak of your powers for that age. Since your knowledge and abilities will have developed and grown, your maturity of thought may have been enhanced, including the way you would have written those entries with hindsight.

Reflection as a nurse is about improvement, and your early reflection entries may have seemed the best you could have written them at the time, but through growth and experience, maybe you look back and wonder if you were self-critical enough, or detailed enough.

Do you regret not pushing yourself or meeting those goals you set?

Maybe you did and you face your next revalidation wondering where you can set new benchmarks.

Perhaps your reflections have indicated you were not happy in your work or life at one time. Maybe they inspire you by remembering how excited the job once made you.

There is much to be gained and little to lose from reflecting. If you want to push yourself to be the best nurse you can be, reflection is one of our best tools for ironing out errors and preventing yourself from becoming complacent.

It can also be an incredibly useful resource in your future career planning. Often it is hard to remember our best examples of development, or times when we did well. One day can often blur into the next in this line of work, sometimes with only a few hours of sleep to separate the shifts. A nurse can use their reflection and personal notes to bring up examples which could go down well in a job interview. That ability to critique your own work and learn lessons is a valued trait.

Have a think about this.

You're a student nurse in your final year of your degree. It's about that time when you begin to think about applying for your first job.

One of the questions asks you about your experience and what you will bring to the role, and you think to yourself, *'experience, I haven't even registered yet, what experience do I have?'*

You're getting concerned now: *'Will they even consider me if I don't have any experience? How do I even complete this application?'*

This is where referring back to your reflections comes in. You look back on the portfolios you have completed as a student. Inside these are little nuggets of gold which you can use as evidence for your job application.

You look at your first-year reflections and find this one:

'It's the night before my first placement in a hospital. I have never set foot in a urology ward before, I even had to google what that meant! I am so nervous. Google is telling me there will be lots of catheter care, I have never even seen a catheter on a real person before, just those mannequins in skills class. What are the patients going to think of me? I feel so under prepared for this placement, I don't even know where to start.'

You read this reflection and think to yourself, *'wow, I was so scared about this experience. As it turns out I loved my time on this ward. It even promoted me to write my dissertation on, 'catheter associated urinary tract infections and how we can prevent them'. If I could go back and tell myself anything, it would be to trust your instincts, the rest will follow'.*

A light bulb goes off in your head: I can show how my experience working in this department prompted me into further research on this topic. My experience here and my further knowledge on the subject will be really useful in the job I am applying for, as there is a lot of catheter care and insertions as a community nurse.

There you have it. Reflection can even help you complete a job application. It just goes to show, looking back on reflections can not only reveal how far you have come, but also sometimes where the light inside you was ignited.

I have just finished a shift in cardiac surgery. Today I observed a patient undergo a coronary artery bypass graft (CABG). I have to admit it but I was dreading today. I am not great with open wounds and a lot of blood. I know that sounds strange, since I am training as a nurse, but I just assumed I would get a job somewhere that didn't deal with that sort of thing on a regular basis. I was so wrong. These surgeons and the nurses are amazing. I saw a nurse called Bindi harvest a vein from the patient's leg to use in their heart. Like, seriously! This leg vein is being moved to the heart and the nurse surgically removed it. I didn't know nurses could do that sort of thing. I am astonished by the skills these people have. This really is life-saving stuff. I can't wait for tomorrow when I am seeing a replacement of an aortic valve; I wonder if Bindi will be there too.

While reflection can be used to document your experiences and interactions with patients and colleagues, which is useful to look back on to assess your progress and development as a nurse, there is also a serious side to reflection. This is the bit that you have to do because you want to continue on the Nursing and Midwifery Council (NMC) register.

Revalidation and Reflection

We have examined revalidation elsewhere in this book, but it is worth exploring the necessary parts of reflection which you will need to submit to the NMC every three years.

The council specifies you must submit five written reflective accounts, in the three-year period since your registration was last renewed or you joined the register.

Each must refer to an example of continuing professional development, a piece of practice-related feedback you have received, and an event or experience in your own professional practice and how they relate to the NMC Code (see Chapter 10).

The NMC's guidance on how to meet their requirements says it encourages nurses, midwives and nursing associates to carry out reflection *'so they can identify any improvements or changes to their practice as a result of what they have learnt'.*

These submissions do not need to be long or academic-style written pieces, the council continues, but they note you must take care not to record information in them, which may identify another person.

That is the written part, but it is the reflective discussion which the NMC says many professionals find most rewarding.

In this, you must hold a face-to-face reflective discussion with a colleague who is also registered with the NMC, known in this instance as your 'confirmer'. The conversation must discuss your written accounts, practice-related feedback and an event or experience and how this relates to the code.

There is another form to complete to mark that this conversation was held, which you are not required to submit, but should be kept safe as part of your records.

I was due to revalidate; my manager, a nurse too, was my confirmer. We have a great relationship and are usually on the same page when it comes to most things in work, that is, except these awful reflections we need to write for our revalidation. I just don't see the point writing my feelings down on a page, I would rather just talk through them, I hate writing and don't know where to even start.

My manager, on the other hand, thinks reflection is amazing; she swears by it, so I ask her for help. She sends me the NMC templates for reflection, I still didn't get the reason for this, but I try anyway, mostly because I have to.

As I start writing, I really begin to think about the whole situation, I write stuff down that I didn't even realise I was feeling. I include some bullet points of things that I feel the team and I could have done differently in future and write in a few ways we could achieve this.

I bring this reflection to my manager, and she's delighted, not only that I actually completed it, but also, as she puts it, 'you've not only reflected on this experience and what you have learned from it, but you have even created a mini action plan with goals'.

I didn't even realise I was doing this, but as I re-read my own words, I can clearly see how invested I am in this and even agree with my manager that I am going to lead on implementing change in this area.

In all, I got a lot out of this reflection. I would totally recommend it.

Theories on Reflection

To learn through experience is not just a simple saying; it is a well-trodden path based on research.

There are three theories below, each with different approaches, which we will analyse in turn. It is very possible these have come up during your studies.

THE GIBBS MODEL

Developed by Graham Gibbs in 1988, this is a cyclical approach, meaning an experience is analysed for reflection and could repeat its cycle if it is experienced again. The core of this being that with experience, lessons could be learnt and key parts analysed, which could come around again to go through the same stages if the event happens a second time.

The first stage is 'description'. Here you are asked to describe what has happened in detail. Think why did it occur, why were you in this moment, what was the outcome, a full description.

Next comes 'feelings'. As the event or experience happened, how did it make you feel, including before, during and after?

Then it's 'evaluation', a weighing up of what was good and bad about what happened, what went well, not so well or indifferent. Was your role a positive or a negative one in what transpired?

On to 'analysis', and this is where the Gibbs Model tries to make sense of it all. Drill down into the experience: why did things go well or not so well, and what is the meaning of it all?

The next stage for Gibbs is 'conclusions' and a summarisation of learning. This is the penultimate stage of this cycle and one where you can assess whether you could have done things differently, for better or worse, for a different outcome.

This leads onto 'action plan' and a judgement on what to do next. Here the individual is asked to map out what they would do differently, but in more specifics, such as what training or skills they need to meet a desired outcome. Is there a way, based on learning and analysis through the previous stages, that slight tweaks in your approach, the circumstances or other people around you, could have made a big difference?

This model tries to find a practical solution to a complex problem, as it centres around a mix of self-analysis of your role and prompting you to find a real solution to what happened.

Gibbs does not want the action plan to be the final stage. His theory is set out in a cyclical form, meaning the next stage after 'action plan' is back to 'description'.

This means, ok, you now have your action plan, your grand design for how to move on and learn from your mistakes or issues in the past, or perhaps it was all a means to improve. Now, when it next comes around, hopefully that action plan has made changes to your description of the experience in cycle two.

One would trust lessons have been learnt through analysis, drawing up conclusions around what happened and why. Now it's time to put that learning into practice. After reflection comes action, and in cycle two there could be a different end result, at least a better one if cycle three ever happens.

Think back to your exam days. Was there a nagging subject you always struggled with to the point where you had written off your chances of a good result before turning the first page? In your studies now, or work life, is there an element of your duties which is so difficult you fear being 'found out' as some sort of nurse fraud because you always have to ask for help, or you simply avoid going near it?

It can be hard to admit to knowledge areas which hold us back but no one knows everything. If there is fear of a subject, confront it; don't give into temptation that it will be fixed by someone else.

Would a little reflection, or self-analysis, to figure out what is holding you back help unleash your potential?

If it doesn't work out the second time, there's always the third time, the fourth, the fifth.

THE JOHNS MODEL

Christopher Johns, like Graham Gibbs, devised his model about nursing, but both have been used in other contexts and different professions. Likewise, there is another cycle involved here, but with a different structure.

First, and it's time to self-analyse again, you are asked to look within. Ask yourself to recall the experience and pay particular attention to the emotions you experienced. This is where, like all areas of reflection, writing down notes about your thoughts and feelings, what it was like to go through in the moment is important. The fresher you write, the more vivid the memories will be.

Here, Johns also asks the user of the model to assess what emotions have been processed in the period since, paying attention to consequences that have arisen.

Next, it's back to a cycle.

Johns takes a different approach to Gibbs, with five sets of questions.

The first, he calls 'aesthetic questions'. This is a focus on feelings and your sensory perceptions. So, what were you doing, how did you react, how did others feel, how did you know what others felt?

Then, it's an area entitled 'personal questions', which is as close to home as it gets. How were you feeling at the time, and why, as well as what factors influenced what you did?

Onto 'ethical questions', and whether your actions befitted your character. Did you have the best intentions in the actions you took? Did your dealings match what your beliefs are, or did other factors come into play that took you away from these, or even become at odds with your principles?

The environment around your decisions features next, with 'contextual questions'. Some of the questions which come into play here are outside influences, did someone or something influence your actions, which you may not otherwise have performed? Have you changed as a result of what happened?

Similar to the Gibbs final stages of conclusions and action planning, Johns finally poses 'reflective questions', using the evidence of your answers from the previous analytical questions to ask what you could or would have done differently. Alongside this, how do you feel now in hindsight? Would another approach have made a difference?

There will always be limitations to using these models, based on the particular circumstances of what you are going through, or wish to reflect upon. In this case, the Johns model may set a series of question prompts to analyse a one-off event but may not help you answer a bigger, deeper question, with more facets.

THE ROLFE MODEL

Gary Rolfe lends his name to a simpler model on paper, but one that poses similar challenging analytical questions. He writes that one should ask three straightforward questions, 'what, so what, now what'.

To take each in turn, 'what' explores a simple definition of the problem at play. What happened, what was your role, what actions did you take, what did you mean to achieve, what was good or bad about the experience?

Then on to the deeper analysis, the 'so what?' What were you thinking as you did what you did? What did you base your actions on and should you have done something different to change the outcome?

'Now what' aims to move your story forward. Once the other factors have been established, what do you need to do to improve the situation or resolve the problem? Are there other issues involved beyond your control and should they be considered in ways to make things more successful next time?

You could be forgiven for thinking these examples are a complicated and time-consuming way to analyse your issues. Perhaps an overly academic way of doing so also if you consider yourself more of a practical person who would prefer a different approach.

The message through all of these models is relatively straightforward, and despite some nuanced differences to their structures, they all aim for a general similar approach. To get to the core of what happened, one must state what happened, lay the evidence out in front of you, then analyse your role and the other factors which came into play. Finally, were there adjustments that could have been made to give a more preferential end result? Then, design a plan for moving forward.

Take this, for example: What happens if you make a mistake, a simple medication error? You administered paracetamol and then realise, *'Oh no, the night staff already gave this patient paracetamol two hours ago!'*

The medication was prescribed twice. That's your first error: You didn't check the stat dose page of the patient's prescription. Your second mistake is actually giving the medication. Your third mistake: not thinking about how this incident has affected you and your patient.

You are really worried. You do everything right, you informed the medical team, even ask advice from the pharmacist, the nurse in charge is aware, the patient is clinically stable, you've documented and informed the patient who responds with, *'That's ok love, at least it's keeping my pain at bay'*.

All of this, and you are still feeling sick to your stomach. You mention this to a colleague, and they suggest you reflect, *'No, sure what good will that do me?'* you respond.

Your colleague insists, telling you, *'Honestly, just try it. I always reflect, and it makes me feel better, as I can get my thoughts down and really process why certain things have happened and how I can learn from them in future.'*

It's a quiet day on shift, and you've just checked on your patient for the seventh time this hour: they are fine. You are free for a little while. You could either clean out the medicines fridge or try out this reflection malarky your colleague is drumming on about.

So you sit down and write the following:

Today I was complacent. I made a medication error. Not a huge one, and the patient is fine; they were actually really nice about it, which was good, but still I made a mistake. I was so stupid. I didn't check the stat doses on the prescription. The bloody paracetamol was prescribed twice, and Ben, the night nurse, had already given it.

I feel sick to my stomach. I know the patient is fine and I have done everything I should to report and document the incident, but I can't shake this feeling.

No one has mentioned it in hours. The patient actually forgot about it until I asked if they were feeling ok while they drank their tea.

I wonder if this stems back to my time in the emergency department as a student. I had such an experience during that placement. One incident stands out though. A young female came into the department. She was unconscious. She had taken an overdose of some sort of illegal drug; I can't remember the name now but I remember my mentor saying it was the usual cocktail for a Saturday night on shift.

This girl couldn't have been more than 19, her whole life ahead of her. Her mother said she had just started university; graphic design was her degree topic. She was apparently so excited and has worked so hard to get there, straight As at school.

Her friend had said that they were at a house party. Someone had brought drugs; they had never taken drugs before but felt pressured to give it a go and a trip to see me and my mentor was the result.

This young girl unfortunately didn't make it. By the time she got to us, the damage was done. I remember being in shock that taking a pill that is so tiny can cause so much destruction. It's crazy to think about it.

Maybe that's why I am so hung up on this medication error; maybe I am so terrified that I might have caused damage and destruction to my patient by being so complacent.

Thinking about the case study above, we can see indications as to why this nurse was finding it difficult to accept her mistake and move on from it. She had, of course, learnt her lesson to always check the stat dose section, and she had done everything right in the aftermath but she couldn't forgive herself.

We can see clearly how her experience as a student has carried through to her experiences as a nurse. Maybe now she can make sense of her feelings and allow herself to forgive her mistake and learn from it.

She will never make the same mistake twice.

Have you seen on social media those progress pictures that people post to identify their health and fitness journeys? Why do you think people post these pictures? Is it to show off? Is it for accountability? Or is it a means to see their progress over a certain timeframe?

It could be all of the above, but that doesn't mean posting such pictures is a bad thing; in fact, it could be quite empowering.

Reflection is quite similar. We can reflect on anything, from finally achieving that skill we have tried so hard for, for so long – *'I finally did it, I finally inserted my first cannula'* – to using it as a means of accountability which allows us to stay on track achieving certain skills, updating training and making sure we are up to date on relevant policies and procedures: *'I have reflected on the changes implemented to help prevent pressure ulcers in my department. Since my last revalidation my ward has successfully introduced a new policy on pressure ulcer prevention from which I have identified several ways in which care has been improved.'*

We also use reflection to help measure our progress as nurses: *'I was looking back on a reflection I did three years ago about providing end-of-life care to a long-term patient on our ward. It brought back so many memories, obviously sad memories as we lost this patient, but also good memories as during this time the patient's family wrote a letter to my manager praising the care I provided to their loved one. This was such an achievement in my career as I had always struggled dealing with end-of-life care due to personal experiences'.*

Reflection, for the compulsory NMC part especially, can at times feel like a chore. You will often want to switch off at the end of a long day, rather than worry about analysing the day's events like it's a post-match studio discussion as pundits pull apart your every move. Let's watch that replay again: what kind of catheter insertion is that? Oh, the manager won't be happy, look at that wound dressing. You get the idea… and I get it, reflection takes energy and time, both of which can be extremely limited in this job. Many negative experiences in particular are ones you want to put behind you quickly, so it can be hard to prioritise making copious notes to act as a reminder.

It is about getting into a habit of making reflections and remembering good and bad experiences. Even creating a note on your phone, or marking it down in a diary each day, two good/bad things that happened. They could be priceless memory prompts for your revalidation examples, and they will also show you how far you have come.

That technique you hadn't mastered a year ago that has now been overcome because you were determined to ask for training… check.

Your nervousness to speak to patients about bad news? We have to do it and you do, but through reflection maybe you devise an action plan to improve your confidence and away you go… check.

Reflection does not have to be limited to the very significant elements of your work. It could be small things, such as tasks you would be embarrassed to admit you need to improve your performance in.

Regardless of your experience as a nurse, your life experience outside of the uniform, your age, your background, whatever, this is a job for continued learning and development. A role to put learning into practice. Nurses rarely have the time to stand still on shift; it is important to never allow our learning to become static also.

CHAPTER 8

What Kind of Leader Are You?

It is fair to say nurses are never far from the headlines, whether it's over our heroic efforts during the COVID-19 pandemic or the times when strike action has been necessary for better pay and conditions. We have also seen our fair share of negative publicity, like the devastating failings uncovered in the Mid Staffordshire Inquiry report by Sir Robert Francis. It is rare to find an evening when healthcare staff do not feature in the headlines, for better or worse.

Healthcare is routinely challenged and reviewed almost daily, at all levels: from scrutiny of the health secretary in the media to clinical managers on wards leading teams on the front line. Everyone in healthcare must play their part to demonstrate effective leadership and management in order for the system to function well and for patients to receive good-quality care.

Ultimately, a breakdown in leadership and poor management will affect the patient.

This chapter is designed to challenge your perceptions of what it means to be a leader in nursing. Sure, there are the managers and people with oversight duties in every trust and organisation. They get paid more, they may even wear a different colour of uniform, and they are people who we look to for support and advice on work-related matters.

They are leaders in the sense that they take responsibility for the actions of their teams or head up projects. But what really makes a good leader or a great manager? In this chapter you will be asked to think about how you would define a good leader in our proud profession in the 21st century.

Ask yourself, what attributes should they have? Do you have it in you to become a leader yourself? Are you already a leader and just don't realise it yet?

One thing is true: no one is born a good leader. When born, an heir to a throne is just another baby. Granted, they may one day be destined for a role that will mark them down in history, but there is no guarantee they will develop the leadership attributes required to command the respect and attention, even affection, of other people.

That has to be nurtured. And if you are at a stage when you question whether or not you could be a leader, remember that there is no deadline. Over time, you may muster skills and a desire to lead. You may even surprise yourself when thrust into a moment when the onus is on you to step up and be counted upon.

Working as a nurse, we know many people in authority. Every trust and organisation has a chain of command, with oversight and management. For every person who gives direction there are others whose job it is to follow it through. Without such order there could be chaos. Defined leadership roles are needed for most organisations to function.

As we begin this discussion, try to think of the leaders you admire. And ask yourself: why do you think of them as leaders?

Were you inspired by a teacher to enter nursing? Do you look up to your parents or guardians as leaders? What about a sporting coach, a historical figure, or a world leader? What marks them out as being different to others?

Perhaps it is their skill with language and conveying a message, or their confidence in decision-making. Maybe it is their coolness under pressure or simply the way they express kindness.

Try to think of three names which we will return to later. Who are the leaders you look up to and why?

1:

Name:

Why are they a good leader?

....
....
....
....
....

2:

Name:

Why are they a good leader?

....
....
....
....
....

3:

Name:

Why are they a good leader?

....
....
....
....
....

Scholars have long debated what it means to be a leader. Indeed, there are reams of academic works on nursing and health leadership.

They focus on the people at the top, those ahead of the registered nurse in the healthcare pecking order: the ward managers, the sisters, the co-ordinators, the chief nursing officer and the health minister. Maybe even the trade union leadership, the journalists and academics who front campaigns and literature.

But what you should consider is: What kind of leader are you each and every day?

If the answer is a quick rebuff to say, 'I'm not a leader and I have no intention of ever becoming one', then you are thinking of the term with too narrow a definition.

So you don't command a team, but have you stopped to think of moments, however fleeting, when you showed little acts of leadership in the presence of your colleagues which had a significant impact on them?

It was a busy day on shift. We all had complex caseloads and everyone had so much to do.

It was mid-afternoon, and one of my colleagues rushed past me in the hallway. She was racing to grab some more intravenous fluids for her patient. I could see it in her face, her cracked voice and the glimmer of sweat on her brow: I knew she was struggling.

I asked her what was happening. She told me about a really sick patient she was caring for. She told me of her concern for her other patients. She felt like she was neglecting all of their needs because all of her time was consumed by trying so hard to save this person's life, along with the medical team.

I had a massive to-do list, but as I stood there with my hand on the observations machine, I thought to myself, I could help. My colleague was an amazing nurse, I looked up to her, but now she needed me.

I wheeled the observations machine into my colleague's bay of patients and started taking their observations without speaking a word to her.

I called upon help for skin checks, ensuring fluid balances and medications were up to date. Soon other colleagues came in to help.

I looked up at my colleague and she mouthed the words 'thank you' to me with tear-filled eyes. She didn't need to thank me. We are a team, we are nothing without each other. I am just happy I helped her so much.

That day was the first time I ever felt like a leader.

(ANN, SENIOR NURSE)

We have all been there, or at some point will be. We notice a colleague struggling. They are confused on their ward round, perhaps distracted by the pressure or things outside of work. We step in and we offer help. We take the initiative and show leadership.

Then there is the time you see a colleague emotional because they have been dealing with a sick patient or they have been involved in a heated conversation with a relative.

You may not head up a department, but allowing your shoulder to catch their tears is leadership, and friendship, and being a good colleague.

That level of empathy is worth the world to the person you are supporting.

This type of leadership appears in a few textbooks. We could even call it nurse comradeship, but it is also leadership. You took charge of the situation and went to the aid of others. You did not refuse or stand idly by; you stepped up.

Those little acts help to define a leadership character, and make no mistake, you will be respected by your colleagues if you show the same level of care for them as you do for the patient.

Have any more names come to mind where people showed leadership around you just because they showed that dedication to helping others?

Types of Leadership

Of all careers, nurses should be pre-conditioned to be good leaders. It is in our nature to take charge of a medical situation and devise plans, keep to strict times for medications, manage bed numbers, make do with staff shortages, explain complex orders in a simple way – the list goes on. We lead at our own level in some way with almost every action.

Telling a patient they have to stop doing something for their health – that's leadership. Changing your tone to console a loved one after bad news – that's leadership too.

Most forms of leadership are judged on a scale.

Laissez-Faire

Or, roughly translated: Let it be or hands-off.

To some, this is not leadership at all, or at least the most ineffective form of it. It is where the 'leader' takes little to no responsibility and passes on decision-making to other members of staff.

Does this remind you of anyone?

Have you encountered people in authority who will shirk from a decision, or create buffer positions around them to shield away from having to make the tough calls?

There will be days when you believe you are better being left alone to work without management breathing down your neck. However, with such a hands-off approach, where is the support network? Can you trust that you can knock on their door for help?

Transactional

What is a transaction? In short, if you give something, you might expect something in return.

In the work setting, this is where the manager, or leader, lays out a task with the employee expecting they will be rewarded for it, whether that is money, time off work, opportunities for development or promotion.

Something given, something received.

Transactional leaders will not look long term like transformational leaders, but more in the short or medium term and work within the existing parameters of their role to achieve success.

Their targets should be fair and achievable for staff, but there can also be a punishment for failure to meet tasks that have been set out.

Something given, something potentially taken away.

Transformational

This is for the long-term thinkers, and some would say the idealists or dreamers.

Those leaders who set out a vision, usually for great change in the organisation, and manage to inspire colleagues to go along with them.

A transformational leader will tend to have strong communication skills and charisma — the type of person who commands attention because of their presence. When they talk, people want to know what they have to say because they have a track record of making a difference.

Consider the example of former Manchester United football manager Sir Alex Ferguson. After the team struggled in his early years, he turned to youth to drive forward success.

He instilled belief that they could make it into the first team ahead of more established and experienced stars, with a set style of attacking play.

The result was the emergence of players such as David Beckham, Paul Scholes and Ryan Giggs, young players who, in their early 20s, began to lead United to immense success.

They were talented footballers, but without the vision and the leadership of Sir Alex, would they have managed the long-term success they did?

Authoritarian

Depending on how you see leadership, this is either incredibly effective or totally ineffective. In a healthcare setting, it is never appropriate.

An authoritarian tells people what to do, often without explanation, and ignores scrutiny. No ifs, nor buts. What they say goes. It is another word for dictatorship and can often go hand-in-hand with bullying.

The result can, in some instances, mean work is carried through extremely effectively. Targets are met and productivity increases. However, at what cost? And how can it be sustainable?

Will the staff be burnt out? Will they eventually rebel because their concerns are not listened to, even on issues about safety or standards?

This can be an isolating job for the leader, who may become suspicious of staff, or seek to keep a few confidants close, and everyone else at a feared distance.

In a caring profession, it is hard to argue that an authoritarian approach is ever conducive to good nursing, at any level.

Leadership Style

This chapter will likely pose more questions than it answers. That is primarily because leadership is a concept. It is subjective.

One person's inspirational leader, who they admire and respect, may, to a colleague, be someone who is too demanding or setting out a vision they disagree with. We are all human with our own opinions.

However, some things we can explore are if there are tell-tale signs that someone is leadership-worthy. Are there attributes you want in your department leaders or are there skills you wish to develop to make yourself leadership material?

The Trusted Leader

Being honest should be a defining characteristic of a good leader.

If you give an inch of doubt to the people you lead that you are not trustworthy, surprise – they will question what you are telling them is true.

Honesty is different from openness.

A lie can be called out, or proven when judged against other evidence, but there is another theory of '*what they won't know won't hurt them*'.

Sometimes it may be necessary for leaders to withhold information or bear the burden of knowing some things to protect those they lead.

Perhaps a plan is not ready for distribution, or some information comes to light which needs more work before it can be shared.

The lack of transparency may cause some to doubt a leader, but there are times when this can be a careful balancing act.

The Communicator

One of the key defining aspects of a leader is their ability to communicate with others. If people do not understand the key message a leader is trying to convey, or feel their directions are open to interpretation, there could be a failure of leadership.

Nurses communicate with each other and with patients constantly. Think about handovers between day and night staff. It is drilled into us to be clear about what work has been done and what is still to come to make sure that nothing slips through the cracks.

Consider those hard conversations with patients about their prognosis, or telling a loved one that they only have a short period of time together. We can learn nursing theory all we want; those conversations are a test of our humanity and compassion.

Fail to communicate well, and nurses risk upsetting or crushing patients in their darkest moments. Developing your ability to speak with others, plainly and with empathy, is arguably one of the most important parts of the job. It is often what you find patients and their families comment on most.

That nurse helped my recovery because they took time to explain my next steps.

The nurse explained the news we feared the most, but we appreciated how open they were and how sympathetic they were to what we were going through.

These are conversations that can test our emotions. Many nurses will leave conversations with patients upset, perhaps remembering what they said for years afterwards. There are good moments too.

A happy interaction to break the good news that a patient can leave the hospital after surgery, for instance, can make this job so rewarding.

There is a nurse's voice which can be utilised here.

The patient and family see you as the person who is key to their understanding of the relevant condition, what they can do to help and what the future prospects look like.

They want to know you are confident in this information, so be confident. They want to know you care, so strike the right tone in this regard too.

At an organisational level, leaders must find ways to break down terms and complicated language in a way which every staff member can understand.

Reflect on the world's great communicators. What do they have in common? How many quotes from Barack Obama or John F. Kennedy's presidential speeches can you recall? Are there sporting moments where the commentator nailed the phrasing of a great moment?

All of them captured a piece of history. They grasped a feeling and turned it into direct and relatable language.

One piece of advice for speechmaking or writing is to shorten your sentences.

Be clearer in the language you use and omit needless words. You want people to listen and read, so set down the thesaurus and speak from the heart. If you have to say it aloud, slow down.

Take your time and emphasise the key words you want people to pay particular attention to. If you dwell on a vital word or pause after an important sentence, the other person's listening ear will perk up.

They will know you intended it to be heard.

Think about these things when you listen to leaders speaking, for example at a trade union congress or a member of your team addressing staff at the morning meeting.

Do they make you wait on every word? Or do you drift off because they fail to be engaging?

The Friend Leader

Nurses work collaboratively, and it is important that we are both honest with our colleagues and communicate well with them.

In many settings, from ward environments to care homes, to list only two, often small teams can often result in close relationships among staff. When you work in such an intense environment, we need to know we can trust each other, so, in many respects, our colleagues become our little nurse family.

That brings many good things. We fight for each other and are there to support each other when it is needed.

However, should leaders be included in that? Or should there be a distance?

Do you want to be on close working terms, or indeed, even friends, with your leaders? Ultimately, they are the people you are accountable to and who could have a significant say in your career prospects or even losing your PIN if the circumstances warrant it.

This is not a point in this book where you are warned about going for nights out with your leaders or doing anything inappropriate, but something you should consider in your career is whether you should have casual conversations with management and get overtly friendly with them.

The balance is for you to decide.

There are many positives to having a good working relationship with those who lead teams, but there are boundaries too that sometimes need to be maintained for that chain of command to function effectively.

The Well-Intentioned Leader

We all want different things from the leaders around us, whether it be clear communication, inspirational messaging or encouragement to do things better.

One thing we should all hope is true about people in positions of leadership is that they are well intentioned, they have decent values and they do things for good reasons.

This again is a subjective matter, but query whether you would rather have your leadership motivated to do the best they can for the organisation, or someone who really could not care, or did not fit well with the ideals of the job.

In healthcare, we can all agree that leaders should prioritise those issues which mean that safety, well-being and prospects of the patient are placed front and centre. That does not mean that staff morale should be overlooked, or planning for resources and staffing to ensure the service can be maintained.

There may be many times during your nursing career when you come to doubt if you made the right decision or if you can sustain the toll that this job can take on your physical and mental health at times.

In those hard moments, consider whether you believe that what you are doing makes a difference.

Think about your own intentions. Are you going through the motions, or does that little nurse fire inside you still burn bright?

If you pursue leadership roles, try to keep that fire going even in times when it tries to flicker.

Challenging Leadership

This is an especially difficult section for those who are just starting out in their nursing career.

The type of conversation you can have with the management is likely to be vastly different than someone who has worked in an area for many more years.

The management knows them, realises their skills base and that what they say may come from more insight and experience.

For you, as a newbie, to raise concerns will likely carry less credibility.

This section exists to say: never be afraid to call out bad practice or to question a leader's decision. Do so with evidence (remember our chapter on evidence-based practice) and back up what you have to say. It is much more likely your thoughts will be taken seriously if there are comparative cases you can point to.

Seek out the advice of your senior colleagues as well.

You will soon know who on your team will be more receptive to this sort of conversation, and indeed, they may back you up in taking on your leaders about a matter.

If you are passionate that something needs to be said, say it. Do not just assume that someone else will raise a matter for you, if you believe in it strongly enough.

In Chapter 10, we delve into this in much more detail as we discuss how to raise and escalate concerns about professional accountability and the Nursing and Midwifery Council (NMC).

What Can I Do to Become a Better Leader?

Every nurse will have different aspirations. For some, their first job was the one and only ambition, the dream role. Others will want to rise through the ranks, believing the sky is the limit, or that their sights rest on a particular job.

If you do seek jobs at a higher level in nursing, it is likely you will be asked about times when you showed leadership. Did you lead a team? Tell us about a time when you were in charge. It can take a while to gain that insight and to build a track record.

One recommendation is to be proactive if you want to be a leader in nursing. Whatever your job, there are only gains to be made from having conversations with the people you admire and whose attitude and attributes you respect.

Have a coffee with them, observe how they manage their time or take meetings. Do they do things better because they've mastered something which you have yet to try?

Most colleagues should be receptive to calls for guidance. It is a little ego boost and a major help to the wider team if, especially as a newer nurse, you are keen to learn more and not just do the minimum required in your role.

There are also countless online resources and books outside of nursing which can help. Check out the courses on offer within your own area of work, or ask colleagues what training they took to take on their role.

Many theories about leadership in nursing are not unique to healthcare. Many of the skills in leading teams, dealing with quarrels and managing resources come straight out of the textbooks of business and other types of management. Take ideas and inspiration where you can find them and see how they might relate to health-care. Think outside the box. That is a characteristic which most great leaders have in common.

Remember Those Leaders You Admire?

During the COVID-19 pandemic, you probably noticed memes or gifs of a nurse under the tagline '*not all superheroes wear capes*'.

Not to brag, but we know this is true: it is hard to do this job without near-superhuman abilities at times.

What this chapter has set out to achieve, however, is to make you think of yourself as a leader too.

Let's ignore the fancy job titles which imply leadership. Be honest and assess the ways in which you show leadership on a daily basis.

At the start, you were asked to list three names of people you admire as leaders and to explain why you believe they deserve to make the list.

As you make it to the end of this section of the book, have any other names come to mind? What about your colleagues, your friends, your teacher? Do you intend to think differently now about what it means to be a leader, or what kind of leader you want to be?

Here we go again. Some space for you to jot down your thoughts.

What are the key things I want to see in the leaders around me?

....

....

....

....

....

Complete this sentence: I am a leader because…

....

....

....

....

....

CHAPTER 9

Novice to Expert: Shaping the Future of Nursing

So you've qualified, you've passed your preceptorship and survived your first six months as a registrant: What now? I know what you're thinking: it's finally time to relax into your role…or is it?

With the introduction of a new programme for student nurses in clinical practice, you now may be required to become a mentor or, what they are now called, a practice assessor, practice supervisor or academic assessor on top of being a new nurse.

But what exactly is this all about?

In January 2019, the Nursing and Midwifery Council (NMC) implemented a new system which replaced the traditional process of mentorship in student nurse education. This change saw the end of mentorship and the introduction of practice assessors, practice supervisors and academic assessors. This new programme which has been rolled out across the United Kingdom has completely transformed the student nurse experience in clinical practice; some of you may have even been students in this new programme.

But what does it all mean for you as a newly registered nurse struggling to find your own feet?

Definitions

Before we start, here are the NMC definitions of the roles associated with the new mentorship process.

The NMC defines that:

1. Practice assessors will assess and confirm the student's achievements for practice learning and recommend students for progression in partnership with the academic assessor.
2. Practice supervisors will supervise students on placements. Any registered health or social care professional can undertake this role. All nurses and midwives should be capable of acting as practice supervisors.
3. Academic assessors will collate and confirm the student's learning and achievement in theory.

According to the NMC (2018), in addition to the changing of the name from mentor to one of the three new roles, there will be further changes in how student clinical practice is shaped and assessed. These changes include the following:

> **BOX 9.1 ■ Changes to Mentorship**
>
> - The term 'mentor' will no longer be used and the traditional role of a mentor will change.
> - The sign-off mentor role will cease to exist in its current form.
> - Practice learning and support of students will officially be the responsibility of every registered practitioner, as stipulated in the NMC Code (2018).
> - The 40% mentor–student contact requirements will be removed.
> - Triennial review will no longer be a requirement.
> - Other registered professionals (non-nurses/midwives) will participate in the supervision of students.

What Does the NMC Say About Practice Supervisors, Practice Assessors and Academic Assessors?

Nurses and midwives who take on the role of practice supervisor, practice assessor or academic assessor must have a current registration with the NMC, can be newly qualified or have many years of experience.

In order to take on one of these new roles, each nurse must firstly be supported by management in order to carry out this additional duty.

Secondly, each individual must also undertake some sort of preparation which should include access to a lecture; this may be in the form of E-learning or in person depending on where you work.

The nurse must also have access to a practice educator who will help to guide and support these nurses through this journey and be there to help answer questions or give advice.

For more information, see Standards Framework for Nursing and Midwifery Education 2019 and Standards for Student Supervision and Assessment 2019.

The reality is that you as a new nurse could be asked to assist with students in your workplace because of the real shortage of available nurses with the recommended experience or training.

If you are asked to assist in a student's journey, you must be prepared to offer support under the NMC Code, but remember, you also have the right to receive support and preparation for this role.

Why Have the NMC Implemented These Changes?

The NMC has taken the decision to reshape the student nurse clinical experience programme in order to deal with various challenges they were made aware of, including the following:

> ### BOX 9.2 ■ Challenges With Traditional Mentorship Programme
>
> - Students were being passed on clinical placements even when their clinical supervisors/assessors had doubts about their performance.
> - 'Benefit of the doubt' or consideration for 'personal problems' led registered nurses to pass students who had not clearly demonstrated competence in the clinical area. If this occurs, registered nurses should contact tutors/appropriate university staff, in writing, as soon as concerns are raised over a student's performance.
> - Inadequate staffing levels and exceptionally high number of students – not enough mentors for students.
> - Students felt they were not gaining appropriate support and training in practice areas due to the shortage of registered nurses with mentorship training.

Why Get Involved Working With Students?

Do you remember what it was like to be a student nurse on placement? Or are you still a student on placement? Do you remember the mentors you had: the good, the bad and the just okay? Think about your experiences and your interactions with these fellow nurses; how did they make you feel? How did these events shape the type of nurse you want to become, or the type of nurse you are today?

Did a bad experience with a mentor change how you felt about approaching certain skills? For example, was a mentor snappy, rude or impatient with you when you were trying to take blood for the first time? Do you now have a fear of doing this particular skill and try to pass this task onto someone else?

It is commonly known that the experiences we have can shape and influence who we become as individuals. Think about that for a second.

Our experiences can leave indents on our subconscious mind which re-merge when we relive similar events or activities. How fascinating is the human mind?

This is why it is so important to ensure the next generation of nurses have positive experiences during their training which will lead them into becoming great practitioners.

We talk so much about providing patient-centred care, and we think always about providing the patient and their families with good, positive experiences, but somewhere in here we need to remember that our experiences count too.

As you know only too well, during our nurse education we spend approximately 50% of our time on clinical placement with the other 50% completing academic classes.

Sure, we learn a lot sitting in stuffy lecture halls listening to someone drone on for two plus hours about the body systems, the 6 Cs and what medications we can't give when and why.

But it isn't really until we are out there on our placements where the real magic happens.

During clinical placements, students get to experience first hand what it is like to be a nurse today. We learn how to develop our basic nursing skills, understand how research and evidence informs and dictates our practice and why we nurses are a breed of our own, even with our own specific language (nursing jargon and abbreviations).

On placements, students learn what areas of healthcare they enjoy working in, what areas they really don't, and some even ignite a passion for specific role or department.

Clinical placement really is where we learn to become nurses and put all the knowledge and training we have gained at university to the test.

During this valuable time, nursing students can learn the tricks of the trade from experienced nurses, finally figure out what all the different-coloured uniforms mean and who really is who in healthcare. Some may even finally master that skill they just couldn't get in the skills lab at university. Clinical placement, despite how hard and tiring it can be, truly is where the student transforms into a nurse.

You're thinking to yourself, 'Yeah I know all of this, what has this got to do with me getting involved with students when I am freshly finished with my training?'

Well, I believe, as a past student, as a past newly registered nurse and as an experienced nurse, that the best people to guide the next generation are people like you. Yes, you, the newly registered nurse. There are excellent seasoned nurses who provide fabulous clinical placement experiences for students, but those of us who have a few years under our belts may forget (as much as we hate to admit it) how it truly feels to be a student walking onto a ward or into a care home for the first time. How vulnerable and scared you feel. But you, fresh out of your student uniform, will remember how it feels like it was yesterday (for some it may even have been yesterday…or today).

It can be difficult for anyone in today's health service to add something else to their to-do list, even if this added something is guiding a student through your day. But is there anything more rewarding than being told by a more junior version of yourself, 'You really helped me today, because of you I was finally able to take blood'?

Let's take a look at something I wrote a long time ago. It is a reflection from my first three months as a registered nurse. The ward I worked on at the time was severely understaffed and extremely busy with complex patients requiring acute care. I was tasked that day with looking after a second- year student nurse called Lisa, as her mentor was off sick.

I was in b-bay today. The bay on the ward I always dread being allocated. I feel bad saying this, as the patients are so lovely, they are just so sick, and I feel extremely anxious looking after them. I sometimes feel like I don't know what I am doing. I count the hours until the end of shift and hope that tomorrow I am allocated in a different, less intense area.

The difference today was I had a student working with me. Second-year Lisa. She is lovely and eager to learn. I remember being so enthusiastic, like her; now I am always stressed and feel burnt out like I am doing a bad job.

Lisa asked if I could talk her through suctioning one of the patient's tracheostomies and if she could do it the next time. The patient was all for this (they are a biology teacher at a local high school and love when they can be used to educate others through their experience).

To be honest, I still have sleepless nights about tracheostomies even though they are so common on the ward. It is just the one thing I really build up a sweat with. But I don't want to disappoint Lisa, or the patient, so I try.

Lisa does a great job; she's better than me first time. She's a natural, and I feel so self-conscious that she's having an awful day with me and that I am not teaching her anything. She really has been a great help and made my shift feel a little more manageable. I hate when students are used as if they are counted in our numbers; I hope Lisa hasn't felt like this today.

At the end of the shift Lisa hands me a note. She said that I should read it when I get home. She thanks me for the day and says she hopes she can work with me again. I'm glad the day is over.

I get home and open the note. This is what it said,

'Hi Joleen, I just wanted to take the time to sit down and thank you for today. I really appreciate how you took me under your wing while my mentor was off. You didn't have to do half as much as you did, especially letting me get so hands on with patients. I can honestly say that in all of my placements some nurses have held back from letting me get stuck in and I felt like they didn't believe in me or my abilities and that made me second guess if I could actually do it, if I could actually become a nurse. Today was the first time I felt like I could do it, that I am a nurse and it's all because of you, your patience and your teaching. You are a great nurse, I can see you doubt yourself but as an outsider I can tell you that you shouldn't; all of the patients today told me how safe they felt and how you made them feel heard. I hope one day I can be like you. Thank you so much, Lisa'

Honestly, I read this and cried. I didn't realise how much of an impact I could have on someone. I thought back to my time as a student and all of the mentors I had, and it hit me: we nurses really do play such a big role in shaping and moulding students, even if we don't realise we are doing it.

There is no doubt that being a nurse is hard at times, and throwing a student into the mix of your hectic day of caring for sick patients, making deadlines and trying to find your feet can seem overwhelming.

But if we don't guide these students and help them through their journey, who will? These students will be a nurse like you one day. They could even be your nurse someday. Wouldn't you want them to know how to do their job with love and compassion because that's what they have been taught, rather than be nervous, rude and under-qualified because no one took the time to help them on their journey?

There were plenty of nurses who took you under their wing; now it's your turn to help these students learn how to fly.

If I haven't convinced you that supporting students is key to your success as a nurse (it keeps you accountable, focused, up to date and passionate), then take a look at the NMC Code; it's also a big part of your job so you are expected to do this.

The NMC Code (2018) states that all nurses must:

9.4. Support students' and colleagues' learning to help them develop their professional competence and confidence.

We must also,

20.8. Act as a role model of professional behaviour for students and newly qualified nurses, midwives and nursing associates to aspire to.

There it is, in black and white: it is your obligation under the NMC's Code to support students.

But Where Do I Start?

Taking on a student in addition to your own case load can be overwhelming and difficult to balance at times, especially if you are new to your role. It will feel like your to-do list is never ending and you are constantly adding to it rather than ticking things off. I get it. I was once that nurse too, but my experience with Lisa just goes to show that if you just try, you might help a struggling student believe in themselves once again.

But 'where do I actually start?'… let's discuss.

GETTING STARTED

My top tip for getting started: stop thinking about students as another task, another thing that is keeping you from completing your never-ending to-do list. Yes, working with students carries a tremendous amount of responsibility, but with that can also come a great amount of satisfaction as you watch your student grow and develop into their best nurse self.

Providing a positive working environment for students can be an invaluable experience not only for them, as this will help them thrive in their own personal learning and development, but it also will benefit us as nurses by keeping us accountable and focused on our own skills and abilities and the decisions we make. This will benefit our patients overall, too.

Get to Know Your Student and Let Them Get to Know You

When I think back to my placements during my own training and the times, I had those little light bulb moments where I had achieved a certain skill, handled a difficult situation well or understood for the first time what the doctors were talking about on the ward round. All of these experiences were with mentors who supported, understood and helped me achieve my goals.

I am sure if you think about your own experiences as a student, you will recognise that the experiences you gained most from, the events where you learned, you grew and you developed were with nurses who took the time to get to know you and your abilities, learning style and your goals for that placement.

This doesn't mean you need to know every little detail about your student's life. You don't need to know their favourite colour or where they would love to vacation, you don't need to become their best friend and share your inner most thoughts; you just need to develop a professional relationship, one where trust and communication are key.

So…spend time with your student and get to know them, their learning style and what experiences they have had previously. Ask them if they have anything specific they hope to achieve on this placement; if they don't know (and that is totally okay – not everyone understands your area of work), then talk them through what you do on a daily basis, explain what skills they can achieve and offer them opportunities to explore other areas related to your chosen speciality. Together, develop a shopping list of everything your student and you both agree is achievable during their time with you.

BOX 9.3 ■ **Think Outside the Box**

Are you a community nurse? Could your student maybe spend the morning at your local GP surgery working with the treatment room nurses? Could they also sit in on a sexual health clinic with the GP or observe what the community midwife or health visitor does? Think outside the box. This doesn't mean handing your student off to other nurses or colleagues every chance you get. It just means you are assisting them in exploring other areas of the health service and what it has to offer. Ask the student to reflect on these experiences and talk through what they have learnt together so you know too if these experiences are actually benefitting students the right way, and if not, then think again about what other opportunities you could open up for your students.

BOX 9.4 ■ **Recognising Learning Styles**

Recognise if your student has any specific learning difficulties and respect that sometimes they may need a little extra help in certain areas. You don't know this person's background or what they have had to deal with, so just as you would with a patient, be professional, be compassionate and be understanding. Communication in these circumstances is fundamental.

Example

In my third year of my degree, I was on a placement in a nursing home. I had a mentor who was uninterested and made me feel like I was causing issues just by being there. This mentor constantly had me work with the healthcare assistants, which was fine for the first few days, as I needed to get to know the routine of the home; it gave me time to develop relationships with the residents and learn their ways. As time went on, I asked my mentor if I could assist in more of the registered nursing duties, i.e. medication administration and wound care. My mentor agreed to let me 'help-out'. So we decided to work together on creating a care plan for a new resident. I completed what had been asked of me and showed my mentor. I was shocked when my mentor started laughing and telling me, *How do you expect to be a nurse when you can't even spell?'* I then apologised and told them that I was newly diagnosed with dyslexia. As a result of my learning difficulty, my mentor told me I wasn't safe to administer medications in case I couldn't read them properly.

How do you feel after reading the case study above? In the box below describe how you would feel if you were the student in the situation.

1.
2.
3.

Now, in the box below tell me three ways you would have handled this differently.

1.

2.

3.

The case study we have just read is my own experience. It is the memories of an experienced nurse, an author, an avid reader and person who has dyslexia but is a safe practitioner who simply has a different learning style…and yes, sometimes can't spell tonsillectomy (did I get it right this time?).

I remember this situation so clearly, not because it was a good experience but because it was a difficult time for me. I had just been diagnosed with dyslexia, something I knew very little about, and I already felt so insecure, and this experience made things so much worse. I began to think to myself if I was good enough, if I actually could make it as a nurse.

It is safe to say I proved my mentor so, so wrong. Please let my experience prove to you that you can and you will do it! We all have different struggles; some of those struggles are visible and others, like mine, are invisible.

If you have a student who has learning difficulties, then talk to them. Ask them what you can do to help them and make their life easier. It might be as simple as changing the colour you print the hand-over on. Using yellow paper makes it a little easier for people with dyslexia to read from. When I worked on the wards, one of my managers always ordered yellow paper and had all our hand-overs printed on this so I didn't feel like the odd one out every morning. It was seemingly a small act of kindness by her, but it made a huge difference for me.

Sometimes all someone needs is a little act of kindness or a chat about their abilities. If a student doesn't feel comfortable or safe discussing their different learning styles initially, at least you have broken the ice, and when they are ready to talk, they know you will be open to listening.

Just one last thing on this: no matter what you face in life, rest assured that if you want to achieve something, you can and you will. Don't let anyone tell you otherwise. Join me in proving how good you really are!

How Do I Manage My Days With a Student?

- If you work in a hospital setting, then include them in the hand-over – ask your student to use a highlighter to highlight or take notes of things they don't understand; then, before you start your day, take some time to go through these areas. You don't need to spend hours working through every point. Simply explain what each thing is and give an example of how this patient is affected. You could then have the student do some research and learning later in the shift. This means the next time they come across certain things, they will have a better understanding of what is actually going on.
- Discuss the basic plan for the day even if that will change – i.e. meetings, visits, clinics or duties/tasks. This will make them feel included and they will be able to use their own initiative when forward-planning their workload.
- Ask the student to bring a notebook and a pen with them to take notes throughout the day about areas they aren't sure about. Maybe you can't explain certain things in the moment, maybe they don't feel comfortable asking questions in front of the patients or other colleagues – whatever the reason, if they have written it down, they won't forget to ask you about it later.
- Allow the student to get involved. If you are taking blood, for example, and the student has completed the theory and practice at university, ask them if they would like to give it a go (of course, with patient consenting). Be with them during every step but don't hold their hand – let the student set up their own clinical space and ask if they need you to check over it; sometimes they will and other times they won't. Get them to talk you through things quickly first, then observe as they carry out the task. If they don't succeed, let them practise again (patient consenting) or at a different time but discuss how they did and praise them for having the confidence to try. Sometimes all we need is a little encouragement to get back up and try again.
- Let the student help with documentation – this is important in our role, and students need to know how to get this right. Maybe use a blank page and discuss what they need to include first – let them draft something up, you 'proofread it', then let them document in the notes. Obviously you'll need to proof

this and countersign too. The content of their notes will show you how well they understand what is going on with the patient. You can both discuss each patient separately too and check off that you have completed everything you need to for that day and plan future care if this is something that is applicable in your area.

- Take breaks together – the student is shadowing you; this doesn't mean they can carry on working and covering you – that is not their job. You don't need to eat lunch together. If you normally like to take a walk alone at lunch, don't let this stop you. Just make sure your student is on break when you are. They are not your understudy.

- Tell the student what you plan to do next and ask them if they would like to help/observe you or if there is something they would like to try to take on themselves. This could be anything from updating the patient notes to helping ambulate patients or responding to email queries; if they feel confident and explain how they plan to carry out said task, give them the independence – but be only an earshot away in case you are needed for support.

- Be flexible. Say you both have planned the afternoon and what you would like to achieve but the student finds out there is something interesting happening with another nurse that they would like to help out with or observe. Then let them do this (obviously if your colleague is accepting). They do not need to be with you all of the time.

- De-brief after shift, and ask them how they feel and what they would like to achieve on their next shift. Ask them to take a look at their outcomes for university and set goals for the next shift – this can be done on shift so the student isn't bombarded with work to do after a long day; let's face it, would you want to go home to do more work? No, then why is the student any different?

- If you are having a busy day and feel overwhelmed, it is okay to tell your student this. To explain that you feel under pressure and you will carry out a certain task this time so you can both catch up doesn't mean you are obstructing the student's learning. This still helps the student to learn because they can observe you. While doing said task, talk the student through it; this helps their learning and yours.

- Give the student appropriate chunk of work to complete independently so you have time and space to move on with time-critical work – always be honest with the student if you are struggling, as this will give them a better insight into what life is really like as a nurse.

HAVE A PLAN

When you know you are expecting a student, plan ahead.

Make a checklist of everything you think the student will need in order to have a successful placement: for example, orientate the student to your area of work and explain the general health and safety regulations including what to do in the event of a fire. Make the student aware of expected break times and the facilities they can use, including the restrooms.

This may seem obvious to you, but what if the student has never worked in a department like yours before? How are they expected to know where the toilet is, let alone what to do if a fire breaks out?

Before you and your student begin any work, take some time to sit down with them and get to know them and what they hope to achieve on their placement. Set goals, some short term and others longer term.

Plan a date when you both will check in to see how the student is progressing and if they have met their target goals for this placement. Plan at least two check-ins with your student during their placement just to make sure they are coping okay. This doesn't need to be a long meeting and could be a quick chat over coffee, but taking the time to talk to your student and asking them how they are feeling might be the difference between them passing this placement with flying colours or struggling to make it through.

My placement involved working with cancer patients, most of them really unwell and at the end-of-life stage. I lost my mother 18 months prior after a long battle with breast cancer, so I really dreaded this placement, as I felt it would bring everything back up for me. I was on to my second week of four when my mentor asked if we could catch up over a coffee to discuss how I felt I was getting on. To be honest, I wasn't doing great; in fact, I was struggling to cope and worried I wasn't going to make it through this placement. I told my mentor how I felt and explained my reasons for this. Her response was amazing: not only did she help develop a plan to support me in practice, but she also put me in touch with a cancer-specific grief consular to help support me through my loss. I can honestly say, if my mentor hadn't been proactive in checking in with me regularly, I would have failed that placement as a result of the stress and anxiety I was feeling at the time.

(RAHIM, SECOND-YEAR STUDENT NURSE)

Below is a checklist I would use with some of my students. You can edit and adjust the checklist to suit your own area of work, but it might give you some tips on how to get started when working with a student for the first time.

Orientation	Initial meeting	Assessments	Check-ins
Explain health and safety including fire safety policies and procedures – be sure to point out fire exits and emergency equipment points	*Meet with your student and ask them what they hope to achieve – set goals for the placement: at least three short-term goals and two long term*	*What experience does the student have? What stage of their training are they at and what do you hope they could achieve during their time with you?*	*Plan an initial check-in, not long into the placement so you can identify and rectify any teething problems that have been established early on*
Give the student access to the local policies in your area of work	*Plan time for the student to shadow you so they can get to grips with the routine*	*Take a look at their skills outcome list and make a shopping list of what the student could potentially achieve while working with you on this placement*	*Reassess goals and how the student is developing – do they need additional support in certain areas? Do you need to reassess goals?*

Orientation	Initial meeting	Assessments	Check-ins
Show the student where the toilet facilities are and explain where they can take their breaks	*Get to know your student – ask them about their previous experience*	*Assess if there is scope for additional experience while on this placement – for example, could you and the student arrange a visit to theatre to observe an operation? Could the student shadow the physiotherapist one afternoon? Think outside the box.*	*Second check-in – give feedback on how you feel the student is progressing and offer constructive criticism if necessary but be positive and encouraging. The last thing you want to do is make the student feel bad if they aren't doing as well in certain areas as expected. Discuss how you can support and develop your student.*
Ask the student if they have any allergies or medical conditions you need to know about. For example, does the student have diabetes and need to store their insulin in a fridge?	*Is there anything you need to know about this student? For example, learning difficulties, travel difficulties or caring obligations outside of placement which may mean adjustments need to be created for this student?*	*Assess the student throughout their time on this placement. Ask them to explain the theory behind the clinical duties they are carrying out to ensure they understand what they are doing and why.*	*Ask the student for feedback on their experience with you – this is always a great way to see how you are doing and identify areas you could improve on too. Plus it's also great preparation for your revalidation.*

What Support Do I Have?

If you continue to feel like you don't have time to give your all for your students, then speak with your manager about what support they can offer you. This may mean a reduced allocated workload or maybe you take time to get caught up without working with the student while they work with another nurse for a little while.

If you don't ask for help, how do you ever expect to get it?

Be open and honest. If you find that you are not able to support students, either because you don't feel you have the skills or because you don't have the time or resources, it is your obligation to speak up.

This is also outlined by the NMC:

13. Recognise and work within the limits of your competence.

22.3. Keep your knowledge and skills up to date, taking part in appropriate and regular learning and professional development activities that aim to maintain and develop your competence and improve your performance.

Your manager will be your first line of defence. You can also take a look at what your union advises you to do in situations where your manager either isn't listening to your concerns or is not in a position to provide you with the support you need as a result of staffing levels and workload pressures.

There is always help out there; we just need to ask for it. My key tip here is: be open and transparent with your student about how you are feeling. You don't want them to feel like this is their fault or that you don't want to work with them. Make sure to let them know this is simply a matter of feeling overwhelmed with the amount of work on your caseload.

BOX 9.5 ■ Hints and Tips

- Spend time with and encourage your student
- Check in at regular intervals
- Have set dates for check-in
- Set goals and reassess during check-in
- Be approachable
- No question is a stupid question
- Be open to questions – they indicate the student is engaging and showing progress
- Give constructive feedback – offer support if the student is struggling, and be compassionate to outside factors
- De-brief difficult situations
- Show that you care

WHAT IF THE STUDENT ISN'T ENGAGING OR FAILING

Tracie is a final-year nursing student and has just started her second-to-last placement with Chris, a staff nurse in Sunny Day Centre for clients with learning difficulties. Tracie wants to be an emergency nurse working in a major trauma centre when she finishes her studies. She has even applied for this post as part of the rolling pre-registration job pool. When this placement came up for Tracie, she was annoyed and disappointed, thinking that she wouldn't learn anything that would prepare her for her future role. On her first day Tracie was late, uninterested and in a mood because she didn't want to be there. Throughout the day Tracie didn't engage with clients or staff, and didn't try to use her initiative to ask questions or help out with daily duties and tasks. Instead, Tracie sat in the corner of the room with her phone. Chris tried repeatedly to get Tracie involved, without any luck.

Chris loves his job; he loves being a nurse and thoroughly enjoys working with students. He was excited to hear Tracie was coming to join them for a few weeks. He didn't expect the impression and reception he received from Tracie on her first day. As the week went on, Tracie's attitude and work ethic didn't change. Despite Chris's best efforts to involve her, talk to her and explain the nature of his work, Tracie's mobile phone took priority.

Chris knew he was trying his best and this was not a reflection on his abilities. He decided to sit Tracie down and have a private, open and frank conversation about her progress. He told Tracie that she was failing this placement and that she was acting in an unprofessional and inappropriate way in the workplace.

Tracie sat up, put her phone down and realised that she needed to stop being grumpy about not having a placement in emergency care. That she needed to make the most of this placement so that she didn't fail.

Following this conversation, Tracie's work ethic and interaction with clients and staff completely changed. She was brilliant and developed strong bonds with everyone, even so that when it came time for her to move on, she left with tears in her eyes.

In the end, all was well, but without Chris taking the initiative and Tracie coming to understand the value in her placement, it could have continued along a disastrous, fractious road. As has been repeated throughout this book, your nursing career is a journey, and until retirement it is hard to pre-determine the exact road you will follow. In Tracie's case, she may well pursue her ambitions, but her single-mindedness has clouded her judgement on the other areas of nursing and that there are skills and fresh perspectives she can gain from this placement and this mentorship which will stand her in good stead. Leaving a placement with tears in your eyes is something many nurses can identify with. We are a family after all.

Chris took the right approach: he identified the problem and sought to mediate in a way which calmed the mood and made Tracie realise there was something to be gained.

When you are in Chris's shoes someday, be sure to orientate the nursing students, engage with them, make them feel wanted and involved. Ask them where they see their future careers. Do not take offence if it is not in your discipline or place of work, but through inspiring and guiding them, leave a good impression that means they will always think fondly of their placement and the people and family they left behind.

BUT WHAT IF THE STUDENT SIMPLY WON'T ENGAGE?

It is your job to protect patients from bad practice, and the student must be failed if they are not safe or competent. In the event that a student is failing, give them every opportunity to achieve and be successful.

Provide them with feedback and identify gaps in skills and knowledge and deal with issues straight away. If another colleague tells you that your student is failing, do not take their word for it; assess this yourself and trust your own judgement. If you need, ask for help from your manager, the placement manager or the university. Give the student the chance to put their story forward; you never know, there might be some circumstances which cause them to be distracted while on placement.

Before you approach your student about their failure, be sure to reflect on the situation first so that you can discuss things with your student with a clear mind. Be sure to give examples about the areas of the student's practice which you are concerned about. Offer support and make plans to move forward, letting the student know that you are still willing to help them.

CHAPTER 10

Professional Accountability and the Nursing and Midwifery Council

Every nurse has the fear. What if I do something wrong? Did I get my medications right? What if I make my sick patient even worse? What if… what if…

For many, accountability and the fear of losing your PIN can be overwhelming, especially if confidence is low, which can happen when you are newly registered, or when there are distractions or short staffing, which can happen regularly.

This chapter is where we will discuss the importance of knowing what we are required to do and why, and how vital it is that we seek support or guidance if we are unsure.

At its core, the Nursing and Midwifery Council (NMC) is not out to get us. They are not a shadowy villain waiting to trip us up.

Take the approach that if you stick by the rules, then you will be able to justify your own actions if you are questioned about a decision.

It will also help you observe if your team is operating with good practices.

Accountability in nursing exists to protect the nurse, the patient and the public's trust that we will act in their best interests.

These high standards are the reason the NMC exists.

Its primary function is to uphold and promote the best practices of nurses, nursing associates and midwives in the United Kingdom (UK).

The NMC's Code is an accountability mechanism you should, or I trust will soon, be very familiar with.

The Code

This is the nursing bible and your new favourite song.

You will never be asked to recite every lyric, but such is the importance of the code, it would do no harm to play it on repeat.

Consider another metaphor while asking what the alternative is: Would our roads be safer without driving tests and the highway code?

Sure, cartoon fans would revel in a real-life Wacky Races, but without lanes to stop us drifting we would lose direction.

Without traffic signals that force us to apply the brakes we could plough head-first into a scene of chaos.

The code provides order and helps nurses to avoid the pitfalls, if we pay attention.

Like many rulebooks, the code has evolved. Each element has been thought about, discussed at length and worded carefully to provide clarity about our roles.

Much of it has been developed because of past events and the need to learn from bad practice to promote the good.

Nursing is such a complex job with increasing demands that the code has had to keep pace, or take a step ahead, to offer protection.

From its introduction, the code highlights that it must be upheld by nurses, nursing associates and midwives: *'Whether they are providing direct care to individuals, groups or communities or bringing their professional knowledge to bear on nursing and midwifery practice in other roles, such as leadership, education or research.'*

Highlighting that the code can be applied in a range of settings, the values and principles *'are not negotiable or discretionary'.*

The code is broken down into four sections, which we will examine a little in turn. This should not be seen as a full debrief on the code. There really is no substitute for reading the document in full.

In addition to the code, there are numerous publications that are important for you to become familiar with which will help develop and support you and your practice. These publications are updated regularly and are available free on the NMC website.

Take a look at:
- Record keeping
- Revalidation
- Raising concerns: Guidance for nurses, midwives and nursing associates
- Guidance on the professional duty of candour
- Social media guidance
- Safeguarding
- Professionalism

Prioritise People

We all know that in nursing, our priority is the patient. They are at the centre of everything we do.

So it's not surprising that the code explains the care of people is *'your main concern'.*

'You make sure that those receiving care are treated with respect, that their rights are upheld and that any discriminatory attitudes and behaviours towards those receiving care are challenged', it continued.

To do this, the code specifies that you should treat people as individuals, avoiding assumptions and recognising diversity and individual choice.

We must not assume that everyone wants the treatment and care we are providing. This doesn't just mean in terms of their medical care; this also involves their social care.

For example:

You work on a busy ward and you're working the night shift.

On your ward the night staff normally wash the patients in the morning before day shift arrive to help ease the morning pressures.

However, you have a patient who likes to sleep in and get washed mid-morning. What do you do?

Do you let the patient sleep in or do you tell them they need to get up to get washed?

Of course you let them sleep in. If this patient doesn't want to get washed in the early morning, that is their right to decline. This doesn't mean they don't get assistance if they need it; it just means things will need to be shifted so that they can get the help they need at a time that works for them and you.

Would you like to be woken up at 6 am to get washed after a broken and restless sleep all while feeling unwell? No, so why would you expect this of your patient?

Nurses must ensure treatment is delivered without undue delay, it added, while they must also respect and uphold people's human rights.

This section also focuses on listening to people and empowering them to share in decisions about their treatment and care.

Scenario One

Nurse: *Joseph, the medical team have decided you are having surgery for your knee arthritis.*

Joseph: *But nurse, I would rather not have surgery; can we not try something else like injections first? My friend has those and they worked for him.*

Nurse: *This is your plan of care, so you need to have it or I have to say you are refusing care and you will go to the bottom of the list.*

Scenario Two

Nurse: *Hi Joseph, the doctor and I have been discussing options for you and your knee arthritis. We have a few options; you could go ahead and have surgery, but we could also try hydrocortisone injections for a little while to see if they help your pain. How do you feel about either plan? Which would you prefer?*

Joseph: *Thank you nurse for including me in this decision about my own care and health. Could you explain a little more about both options so I can make an informed decision?*

Nurse: *Yes, of course I can.*

Which interaction do you feel is more empowering to Joseph?

Which of the two scenarios provides Joseph with respect and allows him to be a part of the decision-making process?

Scenario one ☐
Scenario two ☐

Sometimes this may also mean you have to *'respect, support and document a person's right to accept or refuse care and treatment'.*

'Nurse: But doctor, if they don't accept this blood transfusion, they could die!

Doctor: I know, nurse, but this person has the right to decline any treatment, including that which may save their life.'

Part of being a nurse is to recognise that everyone has the right to live how they want to. It is not your job to interfere with people's decisions, even if you disagree with the outcomes. As long as the patient has capacity to make their own decisions, the decision about accepting or declining care is their own, not yours.

Every person is legally competent unless a suitably qualified practitioner has deemed otherwise.

Everyone will have the competence to make a decision, though this can vary based on what the situation is. Some people may have the capacity to decide if they want to have a shower or eat a certain type of food for dinner, but they may not have capacity to consent for surgery.

Everyone is different, and we need to look at the bigger picture when nursing any patient and adjust our care and treatment based on what the patient wants.

It is highlighted that nurses must meet the changing needs of patients *'during all life stages.'*

This can mean recognising and responding with compassion to those who are in the last few days and hours of life, as well as acting *'as an advocate for the vulnerable.'*

'Nurse: Manager, I think my patient may be experiencing financial abuse. This lady has dementia and isn't aware of her finances, I have my suspicions as this lady does not have clothes that fit, her shoes have holes and she is underweight. She lives with her grandson who is listed as her main carer. She has a good pension coming in and I am aware her mortgage was paid off years ago. I am concerned she isn't actually receiving her pension and her grandson is stealing from her'

'Manager: You are right to report this, we need to investigate. This lady needs us to be her voice if this is happening'

Nurses must act in the best interests of people at all times, which can include obtaining properly informed consent or telling colleagues if you have a conscientious objection to a particular procedure.

Consent can be given in multiple ways. Verbally, in writing or simply by co-operating with the given task.

For example, you are chatting with your patient about the weather while assisting them into bed. You next task is a blood pressure reading. You continue your conversation and simply hold up the blood pressure cuff, the patient puts their arm and you obtain their blood pressure.

You haven't specifically asked for their consent to carry out this task, but their cooperation displays that they are agreeable, so consent has been gained.

What if there is an emergency, the patient is unconscious and you can't gain consent. What do you do?

You are expected to do whatever is needed in order to preserve life. However, what if this patient has refused certain investigations or interventions previously; do you take this as your opportunity to carry them out? No! You can't ask the patient this time, but you should know in your heart that they would decline this treatment or intervention, so discuss this with the wider team.

On occasion, some people will leave advice with family or friends, or will have left a document which indicates their intentions in certain situations, like their wishes on end-of-life care and organ donation. This will of course need to be considered when planning any interventions or care, and you should always seek advice from someone more senior before you do anything.

Privacy is also outlined in the code as owing a *'duty of confidentiality to all those who are receiving care'*.

Familiarise yourself with your local policies on data protection, but the key thing to remember here is always protect your patient's dignity and privacy whether that be during personal care tasks or if they ask you not to share their diagnosis with family. Always uphold the patient's wishes and their dignity.

Think about how you would feel if you were in their position. Would you want your life story on broadcast to every Tom, Dick and Harry on the ward, or would you prefer your information is protected and is on a need-to-know basis?

I know which I would choose.

There is a reason why sensitive health information is referred to as sensitive; it is because it is deeply personal. The protection of data and a patient's information has always been a priority in health care, but there is added scrutiny today because of the Data Protection Act (2018). This legislation established rules for how organisations and the government disseminate and keep records, preventing unwanted access, keeping the information on file for only as long as necessary and placing limits on how it is used.

Consider if it was your health information or your family. You would want the medical professionals involved in the care to know what they need to know of course, but it is nobody else's business, nor should there be a risk that it could be shared or used for other purposes.

Your employer may have protections built into your day-to-day work for this. Many people who work in health care will have secure email addresses or online systems which do not allow information to be exported or be susceptible to hacking.

It is an issue to be taken extremely seriously, as government guidelines state that a heavy fine or compensation could be imposed if personal data is misused.

Training should be offered by your employer about record keeping and data protection – consult with your manager about how data protection will affect your role.

Practise Effectively

Alongside informing nurses they must deliver care to the best of their abilities, this part of the code notes the importance of learning lessons.

'You must reflect and act on any feedback you receive to improve your practice,' it notes.

It is a section which urges nurses to practise going by the best available evidence, while communicating clearly in *'terms that people in your care, colleagues and the public can understand.'*

Nurse 1: You have a haemopneumothorax, so we need to insert a chest drain.
Patient: I don't understand, what does that mean?
Nurse 2: You have a collapsed lung and there is also some blood in your collapsed
    lung. We need to place a drain into your chest so we can treat this.
Patient: I understand.

This is an area touched upon in other chapters in this book, with the code confirming how the use of both verbal and non-verbal actions *'to better understand and respond to people's personal and health needs.'*

Nurse to non-verbal patient: Can you point to me which face describes how you are feeling? (Nurse shows patient the Wong-Baker FACES Pain Rating Scale which allows a patient who is unable to communicate verbally to tell the nurse how they are feeling by selecting a face which best describes their pain.)

One must work co-operatively, the code continues, respecting the skills and contribution of colleagues.
You must also be mindful of how to support colleagues *'who are encountering health or performance problems.'*

'However, this support must never compromise or be at the expense of patient or public safety.'

Practising effectively is an element of the code which also focuses on the need to keep clear and accurate records, making sure they are dated and kept securely.
Also, it is vital to do so *'at the time or as soon as possible after an event'.*
As the saying goes, if it hasn't been documented, then it hasn't been done and so true is that statement in nursing. Take this, for example: Would you give a patient their medications and not sign you have done it? What could happen? The nurse coming in after you would see the blank prescription and think you've missed it. What if the patient can't tell you *'the morning nurse already gave me that injection.'* You would probably try to get a stat dose prescribed and give the patient the medications to ensure they haven't missed out… or in actual fact the patient gets a double dose.
So if you wouldn't miss documenting vital things like medication administration, then why wouldn't you document your experience with your patients? What has their day been like have they consented to treatment or declined assistance with personal care? Did you have a conversation with their family member who raised concerns about their home situation or about their ability to manage on their own upon discharge?

Documenting our interactions with our patients is a vital component to providing gold-standard care. The nurse or doctor who takes over after you can read your notes and see what type of day that patient had. They can read that you have already tried on multiple occasions to assist the patient with their insulin but the patient outright declines, explaining why this patient's blood sugar is now creeping up into dangerous territory.

Our documentation is so important, I could honestly write a whole book on it. In fact, when I used to work on the wards, my colleagues used to joke with me when I said, *'I am just off to do some notes now'*… they would laugh and say, *'You're off to write your book you mean'.*

I have seen first hand how documentation has been used as evidence in disciplinary meetings against other staff. How their records were pulled from years prior to investigate if, in fact, the nurse did raise the concern on multiple occasions that the patient had expressed thoughts of life not worth living.

It really can be the difference between proving that you have done all you could for this patient or giving the prosecution a means to say, *'Well, nurse, it doesn't appear that you had expressed a need for mental health services to review your patient. There is no clear evidence you even had this conversation with anyone – it's your word against theirs.'*

Preserve Safety

A key part of preserving safety is knowing when your personal alarm bells should ring, as well as when you see risk in the actions of others.

The code describes this by urging nurses to work within the limits of their competence while exercising a professional duty of candour, and raising concerns immediately if they believe patient or public safety is at risk.

When the code says to work within one's own competence limits, it means asking for help to carry out actions and to make timely referrals to other practitioners.

This includes advising on, prescribing or administering medications *'within the limits of your training and competence, the law, our guidance and other relevant policies, guidance and regulations'*, the code specifies.

It also means to *'take account of your own personal safety as well as the safety of people in your care'* and to complete the necessary training before carrying out new roles.

Where other sections of the code explore making patients aware of their treatment plans, this portion on preserving safety notes that you should be open and candid when mistakes have been made.

Act immediately, explain fully, apologise and document actions formally.

This will help to rectify matters *'so they can be dealt with quickly,'* the code continues.

Always offer help and *'act without delay'* to raise and escalate concerns if you believe there is a risk to safety.

This extends to the care of people who you believe could be vulnerable or *'at risk from harm, neglect or abuse.'*

As part of this protection, nurses also need to be familiar with the laws and policies about caring for vulnerable people.

Promote Professionalism and Trust

'You should be a model of integrity and leadership for others to aspire to.'

This is how this section is introduced as it tells practitioners to uphold the reputation of their profession, which in turn should *'lead to trust and confidence'* from patients, colleagues and the wider public.

This section directs nurses to stay objective and maintain professional boundaries, to not express personal beliefs in an inappropriate way, to act as role models for students and the newly registered, and to use all forms of communication, including social media, *'responsibly'*.

More on this a little later in the chapter.

There are other potential pitfalls mentioned in this section, including acting with honesty over financial dealings, including with people in your care. Never ask or accept loans from people in your care or anyone close to them.

Refuse *'all but the most trivial gifts, favours or hospitality'* also, as this *'could be interpreted as an attempt to gain preferential treatment'*.

Sections 21.5 and 21.6 also demand that you do not use your job title *'to promote causes that are not related to health'* and to only co-operate with the media when appropriate, ensuring you protect the confidentiality of people receiving care.

This important section concludes by outlining how nurses must co-operate with investigations and audits, respond to complaints and provide leadership to make sure people's well-being is protected.

This involves supporting staff you may be responsible for to follow the code at all times.

Social Media

The chances are you have, or have had, social media accounts. They can be an incredible resource to stay in contact with friends and family; also an opportunity to make new connections, join new groups and learn about the world.

But – and this may sound obvious – the risk of losing control of your personal data, privacy and the potential to be exploited is real.

The NMC has a section on its website dedicated to social media: https://www.nmc.org.uk/globalassets/sitedocuments/nmc-publications/social-media-guidance.pdf

If used responsibly, the council says, social media can 'offer several benefits' for health professionals.

This includes:

- Building and maintaining professional relationships.
- Establishing or accessing support networks and being able to discuss specific interests or research areas.
- Being able to access resources for continuing professional development.

The NMC Code's specific nod to social media comes as follows: *'Use all forms of spoken, written and digital communication (including social media and networking sites) responsibly.'*

This may not go into detail yet, but as the social media guidance elaborates, *'nurses, midwives and nursing associates may put their registration at risk, and students may jeopardise their ability to join our register if they act in any way that is unprofessional or unlawful on social media'*.

Here is where the NMC explains what is meant by bad practice on social media. Such is the risk from social media use to your registration and your very right to be a nurse, and I believe it is important to mention these word for word:

- Sharing confidential information inappropriately
- Posting pictures of patients receiving care without their consent
- Posting inappropriate comments about patients
- Bullying, intimidating or exploiting people
- Building or pursuing relationships with patients or service users
- Stealing personal information or using someone else's identity
- Encouraging violence or self-harm
- Inciting hatred or discrimination.

Social media popularity has grown exponentially over the past decade, bringing with it the need for new guidance. Expect this to continue to change and grow.

An innocent 'add friend' from a patient online could lead to inappropriate connections with them or a dropping of the guard if lines are blurred.

A throwaway comment you give on a news story could land you in bother too if it's seen as bringing your job into disrepute.

Even if you do not explicitly say you are a nurse on social media, many people will know this, and you may never know the moment a remark outside of work could lead to an awkward conversation with management when you next clock in.

The NMC Code asks professionals to remind others of their requirements, and to raise concerns.

It is always advised to think twice before airing opinions or sharing information if it could cause difficulties in your job, whatever the profession.

The official NMC advice: Be informed, think before you post, protect your professionalism and your reputation.

Whistleblowing

'I saw people dying in undignified situations which could've been avoided, it's like no-one cared.'

(CHRIS, NURSE WITH 6 YEARS' EXPERIENCE WORKING IN AN ELDERLY CARE UNIT)

'I raised the alarm with my manager about the unsafe staffing levels and was told to fill in an incident report form…I did but who actually reads them? It's like my written concerns vanished.'

(JOE, NURSE WITH 3 YEARS' EXPERIENCE WORKING IN MEDICAL ADMISSIONS)

'I was told… "this is how we do things here"…even though how they do things is completely inappropriate and undignified.'

(PEARSE, MANAGEMENT STUDENT ON PLACEMENT IN A NURSING HOME)

'Patients were left with their meal trays on the table in front of them but no one would assist them to actually consume the food.'

(HAYLEY, NEWLY QUALIFIED NURSE IN A STROKE UNIT)

'I realised it was time for me to leave this job when I saw the nurse shout aggressively at that little old man because he was incontinent, it wasn't his fault… other staff had refused to take him to the toilet as "it wasn't that time"…how can people be so cruel.'

(HARVEY, EX-NURSE WHO LEFT THE PROFESSION AFTER WITNESSING SO MANY DISTRESSING INCIDENTS IN HIS 6-YEAR CAREER)

Take a look at the statements above again. How do you feel? Disgusted? Horrified? Sick to your stomach?… But what would you do? No, really… what would you do if you were a nurse working in these conditions, with these people as your colleagues?

Would you think this is acceptable practice? Would you think, 'Well at least I treat my patients well?' Or would you… whistleblow?

All employers within health care should have a policy on whistleblowing. In its purest sense, this is calling out bad practice and saying enough is enough. In health care, it may be witnessing an individual at fault or an entire unit which is ineffective or breaching regulations. It could be bullying, it may be witnessing something illegal; you could even find that someone has been stealing.

There are many different topics about which people may feel the need to raise concerns. Some common areas can include the following:

- Abuse of a patient, their family or a colleague
- Discrimination, racism or sectarianism
- Illegal practices such as theft or fraud
- Breaching the confidentiality of patients
- Inappropriate relationships with patients
- Issues surrounding bad practice including poor health and safety procedures.

It can be a terrifying prospect to call out the bad practice of others, especially if you fear that little will come from your endeavours and it will be you who is left to work in an environment where others know you appealed against them, or suspect it was you who blew the whistle.

In December 2021, *BBC News* reported that a doctor at West Suffolk NHS Foundation Trust felt as if she was going to lose her career after management asked her for fingerprint and handwriting samples as they tried to identify a whistleblower. The doctor said the experience left her feeling ill. An independent report found management's approach to be incendiary, with the trust's leadership having to apologise to the doctor and other staff for their conduct.

In an ideal world, management would take complaints and whistleblowing on board, and act on it. However, in some cases there is that fear that speaking out could prompt a backlash, and a suspicious work environment. It is an intimidating prospect to raise concerns. However, there are ways you can be protected and your identity hidden from management.

Employers should have policies that allow you to make confidential statements so matters can be investigated, without it being traced back to you. This can take time and special care to ensure your anonymity. It is worth considering: What is the alternative to not speaking out? Could the bad practice continue, or get worse, through inaction? No one really wants to be a whistleblower, but it is because of whistleblowing that people in authority are held accountable, and people who are unsafe are taken away from the patients whose well-being depends on receiving good care.

You may feel a duty to yourself and your own conscience to become a whistleblower, but think of public safety also. There is a bigger picture within nursing. Sadly, not everyone will aspire to the high standards which they should in this profession. Perhaps if that is the case, they forfeit their right to be a registered nurse.

It must also be remembered our legal duty, under the NMC Code. We are obligated to whistleblow and highlight bad practice. It is spelled out very clearly in the document which is our fundamental rulebook. As a result, no nurse should fear that speaking out is wrong; it is what we are meant to do.

Have you ever heard of the Report of the Mid Staffordshire NHS Foundation Trust (2013), better known as the Francis Report? Well, if you haven't, this is some essential reading for anyone entering the profession. This report brought to light the horrific cases of abuse, neglect and trust failings in one Mid Staffordshire NHS Foundation Trust Hospital. Some findings from this report include the following:

- Patients became malnourished – no assistance was given with eating to patients who could not feed themselves and water jugs were left out of reach.
- Privacy and dignity, even to those dying, were not provided.
- Patients were denied assistance with personal hygiene – patients were left in their own excrement and soiled bedclothes for long periods.

The list goes on…

You may be thinking: How can people who enter into a caring profession show a complete lack of basic and fundamental care?

Take a look at Linzi's story:

'It was my first week on the job, really on the job as a fully fledged registered nurse; I was thrilled, my family were so proud. I had finally made it. After all those years of writing essays, studying for exams, the long days and nights on various wards, care homes and in the community, I had done it. I had achieved everything I had always wanted, so why did my world come crashing down? Why did I find myself surrounded by other nurses, some with over 20 years of experience and some new like me all providing unsafe, unevidenced and undignified care, was this nursing? Was this what I was supposed to be doing? This was my job; I was being paid to be here, so what should I do?'

Speaking Up

Not every incident of whistleblowing needs to be a big dramatic investigation or formal procedure. Sometimes we can call out smaller elements of bad practice with a quiet word. Have you seen someone fail to wash their hands when they should have, or use the phrase 'sure the patient is light, let's just lift them up the bed' when they should really be using a sliding sheet? Maybe they've administered a medication but failed to check a patient's identification. Mistakes, or bad trends in practice, can happen. They shouldn't, but sometimes they do. With a quiet word to the individual or their supervisor or manager, bad practice can be nipped out before it becomes a deeper issue.

These examples could also be referred to as cutting corners. We could compare it to the little habits drivers develop. The heightened alert of checking every wing mirror before a manoeuvre or holding your hands at '10 and two' to mimic a clock face in your grip of a steering wheel are things you should do and will do to pass a driving test. However, most drivers let some of these things slip a little as time goes on. In life, we develop bad practice; we are only human. The trick in this profession, similar to your time on the road, is to remember there are lives at stake. Bad practice cannot be tolerated and needs to be called out.

Speaking up does not always mean speaking up against your colleagues; it can mean speaking up against management and those in higher positions. It can also mean speaking up against patients and their families too.

Much of the NMC Code and the rules we follow as nurses has originated as a result of instances where bad practice has been called out and new guidance was needed to improve our standards and improve our care. This will continue to change and evolve, but one thing will remain: If you witness bad care, it is your duty as a nurse to take the plunge and stand up and speak out.

CHAPTER 11

The Dreaded Revalidation Process

Revalidation…the process to ensure I am a safe and effective practitioner…and to look back and reflect on how far I have come or consider areas which I could improve on

(Leigh, Senior Nurse Approaching Second Revalidation)

You may have read the title of this chapter in disbelief, asking yourself, 'why in a newly registered nurse's handbook are we discussing something I need to do in three years? I can barely think about three days from now at this stage.' Well… yes, your feelings may be totally understandable, but do you remember how fast three years of uni versity went? Do you remember thinking, 'I'm on my first placement of first year, I have so much to learn, but I have time to do it.' Do you also remember feeling like that was yesterday? Well, the next three years of being a new nurse will go just as fast…really, take it from experience.

Revalidation isn't an essay we can have an extension on or an exam we can repeat. This is real life, and there really aren't any allowances here for missing the deadline. You either make it or suffer the consequences of not.

I don't want to scare you here and make you think like you need to complete your revalidation portfolio tomorrow. Instead, I want to make you think each time you complete a new skill, receive feedback from patients or co-workers, or attend training and events related to your practice: 'Could these things help me towards completing my revalidation?'

You'll be doing all of this stuff anyway, right? So why not make things easier for future you?

Throughout this book I have added notes here and there and suggested how certain things we have discussed would work well towards your revalidation. We have explored ways in which you can not only get the most out of your first steps as a nurse but also learn how to achieve and enhance your current skills and how to obtain more.

Now, it's time to put some of those hints and tips to the test and find out how to actually use them when you come to complete your revalidation.

The process of revalidation helped me realise how far I have come in my career, gathering all of the information reminded me of all the training I have completed and looking back at my reflections from my first year as a nurse showed me that I am constantly improving and advancing my skills and abilities

(STAFF NURSE ALISON, INTENSIVE CARE UNIT, FIRST REVALIDATION)

In 2016, the Nursing and Midwifery Council (NMC) introduced a new framework for all nurses, midwives and nursing associates in the United Kingdom (UK) (we will look at nursing associates briefly at the end of this chapter). This new framework is known as 'revalidation'.

Revalidation is the process where nurses, midwives and nursing associates are required every three years to demonstrate that they remain fit to practise safely and effectively.

Revalidation is compulsory in order to renew your registration; there's no hiding from it, so keep reading!

The Requirements

According to the NMC (2022), each practitioner must:

- Complete 450 practice hours in their role, or 900 if renewing as both a nurse and midwife
- 35 hours of continuous practice development, including 20 hours of participatory learning
- Five pieces of practice-related feedback
- Five written reflective accounts
- Reflective discussion
- Health and character declaration
- Professional indemnity arrangement
- Confirmation.

Revalidation for me is a way in which I can demonstrate that I am a safe and efficient practitioner and that I use the NMC code in my everyday practice.'
(COMMUNITY NURSE LOUISE, SECOND REVALIDATION)

It is important to know that revalidation is not about making an assessment of your fitness to practise; it is about promoting good practice across the whole population of nurses, midwives and nursing associates, as well as strengthening public confidence in the nursing and midwifery professions (NMC 2019).

But what does revalidation help me to do?

- Revalidation helps me to be accountable for my skills and abilities and reflect on areas where I have done well and areas where I could improve by reviewing feedback from patients and/or colleagues. This will provide me with a self-confidence boost or prompt me to rectify areas I can improve on.
- Revalidation helps me to reflect and think about the type of nurse I am and what type of nurse I want to be as my career progresses – this helps me to consider if there are actions that I need to take to ensure I get to where I want to be.
- Revalidation gives me the reassurance that I am a safe practitioner and that I am able to provide effective care for my patients.

It is more than just filling out your certificates; it's a resource for you to keep as you go through your career. One way to manage your revalidation is to keep an updated portfolio which you add to regularly, meaning when it actually comes to completing your revalidation, you have three years of training information, reflections and feedback all in one place.

YOUR PORTFOLIO

Your portfolio is for you. It is your little reminder of how far you've come in the past three years. It contains all of your achievements, reflections of your practice, and feedback from those you've cared for and worked with. It's all about you….so make your portfolio suit you and your lifestyle.

You do not need to create the next masterpiece; you aren't Picasso.

Your portfolio doesn't need to look perfect with colour-coordinated pages and pristine handwriting. As long as the end result meets the requirements of the NMC, you can be as creative or as bland as you like.

If you are like me and like to keep things simple, then the option of having a revalidation notebook may interest you. The revalidation notebook is a book that I keep in my locker at work. I take this notebook on training courses with me and add dates, times and a little reflection on what I learnt or how I felt the training went. I don't spend long doing this, only five minutes or so.

I often write in it during my break or at the end of the shift, like a little journal. I reflect on situations if I have had a particularly hard day or celebrate with myself if something really good happened. Sometimes I will even scribble if we had some ad hoc training on shift…or if a colleague taught me a new skill or if I taught them. Whatever it is, I document it here. It is my safe space to get my thoughts onto a page, so when I leave work, I leave them there too.

At the back of this notebook there is a little pocket. This is where I keep thank-you cards or emails from patients and colleagues with feedback about my practice. If I have received verbal feedback, I usually type up this interaction quickly or scribble it on a page and slide this into the pocket also.

I date and time-stamp everything, so when I look back, I can not only remember when this happened but also keep track of what is recent (as in within three years) and what isn't.

When I get some free time, I take my notebook out for a coffee (yes, I go on a coffee date with my notebook). I open a Word document with the NMC's templates already copied in and add things from my notebook to this. I use a red pen to tick things off as I go to make sure when I come back to it again, I don't waste time duplicating things.

I try to do this every six months or so around the same time when I know some of my mandatory training needs to be booked in for a refresher. This keeps me up-to-date with everything I have done, so when it comes to my revalidation, I am basically finished without any stress, and I always know when I need to update my skills so they don't lapse.

There is nothing worse than the feeling of realising a particular skills update time has lapsed and you need to complete the whole course again, rather than a quick refresher (hey there, Intermediate life support, I see you).

You can make this more graphically pleasing by using folders, page separators and colour if you want. I have tried this in the past; it did look good and made me feel really organised. However, what I found was, I spent more time worrying about having the perfect colours and the most pleasing layout that I neglected the actual content.

Sure, when it comes to your revalidation, you need to print everything off and put it all into a nice, crisp folder. But…if you have everything there already and your hardest job is hitting print, then, my friend, you will feel so good.

Recently, a friend and I were discussing reflections and revalidation. He mentioned he felt a little exposed at times by including certain reflections in his portfolio.

I just don't like the thought of my manager knowing my inner most thoughts about how I feel about certain things. I reflect regularly and like to be honest but sometimes when I think about sharing these reflections with others, it sends shivers down my spine.

I asked him why he felt like he had to share these reflections at his revalidation. Could he not summarise them and that's what he showed to his manager? He could leave out some of his personal thoughts and focus on the moral of the reflection.

You don't need to include everything. Yes, this portfolio is yours to include what you want, but that doesn't mean you need to share everything. Reflect until your heart's content, write your personal thoughts, get those bad days and hard experiences off your chest and onto paper, but… when it comes to sharing your portfolio with your confirmer, remember to review and edit what you want others to see.

The whole purpose of the revalidation process is to see your personal growth, to reflect on the good, the bad and the ugly. In our line of work, we all need to process our experiences so we can carry on being the best nurse we can.

You will continue to grow, advance and achieve every day. Some days may feel like you've taken two steps forward and 10 steps back and that's ok. That's normal. Don't be too hard on yourself, be patient and remember revalidation and the NMC aren't the enemy. They are in place to support you, so take the help. You aren't the last solider standing. You have an army all around you. We are all on the same side.

There are numerous outlets for support and assistance with revalidation, most of which can be found on the NMC website: http://revalidation.nmc.org.uk/welcome-to-revalidation/index.html

You can also benefit from talking with your manager or your colleagues about what worked for them when they began to gather information for their revalidation. The Royal College of Nursing (RCN) also have great advice, hints and tips on their website: https://www.rcn.org.uk/professional-development/revalidation

The key point of revalidation is to make practitioners think about and reflect on their practice with the purpose of helping to ignite the desire and enthusiasm to improve, advance and refresh their skills and knowledge. It's not as scary as it all sounds… really, it's actually a pretty rewarding experience.

Before I revalidated it was initially quite daunting, but as I started I found it a really positive experience which helped me develop confidence and emphasise how the code really does underpin everything we do as nurses. Overall it was a positive experience which really makes me think about my practice and how I can continue to become better

(JOHN, WARD MANAGER IN MACULAR CLINIC, SECOND REVALIDATION)

The NMC gives you a basic outline in the form of templates for how you might organise your portfolio. These templates can be found on the NMC website ready to download and edit.

So… let's take a look at what you actually need to do in order to complete your revalidation.

BOX 11.1 ■ Practice Hours

So the first step in revalidation is completing the correct amount of hours as stipulated by the Nursing and Midwifery Council (NMC), which are:

- Nurse: 450 practice hours required
- Midwife: 450 practice hours required
- Nursing associate: 450 practice hours required
- Nurse and Specialist community public health nurse (SCPHN): 450 practice hours required
- Midwife and SCPHN: 450 practice hours required
- Nurse and midwife (including Nurse/SCPHN and Midwife/SCPHN) or nursing associate and nurse: 900 practice hours required (to include 450 hours for nursing, 450 hours for midwifery, 450 hours for nursing associate)
- If you are renewing three registrations, say you're a nurse, a midwife and a SCPHN, then you will need 1300 hours (wow, that's a lot of hours – let's stick to being the newly registered nurse for now).

If you have fewer hours than what is required, you may need to discuss a return-to-practice programme with the NMC, but before you freak out, thinking '*450 hours is a lot of time working*'. …. Yes it is, but remember it's over three years! Visit the NMC website for more information and what happens if you require time off for maternity leave, etc.

The NMC recommends you use their templates when completing your revalidation. You don't have to and could create your own, but why would you give yourself the extra work when it's already outlined for you?

Let's look at an example:

Michelle is a nurse who is approaching her first revalidation since qualifying in 2019. This is her practice hours log.

Dates:	Name and address of organisation:	Your work setting (choose from list above):	Your scope of practice (choose from list above):	Number of hours:	Your registration (choose from list above):	Brief description of your work:
Start date: 29/09/2019 Revalidation date: 01/09/2022.	General Hospital, 1 Sick Lane.	Clinical/ Hospital based setting.	Direct Patient Care.	5400 hours over 3 years.	Nurse.	Direct patient care in a ward-based hospital setting.

Can you see how it's broken down? When you've done this bit, you've achieved step one; wasn't that easy? Now let's look at step two…

CONTINUING PROFESSIONAL DEVELOPMENT

Here is a section from the NMC website. Read it carefully….

You must have undertaken 35 hours of continuing professional development (CPD) relevant to your scope of practice as a nurse, midwife, nursing associate or combination in the three-year period since your registration was last renewed, or when you joined the register.

Of those 35 hours of CPD, at least 20 must have included participatory learning.

You must maintain accurate records of the CPD that you have undertaken. These records must contain:

- The CPD method
- A description of the topic and how it is related to your practice
- The dates on which the activity was undertaken
- The number of hours (including the number of participatory hours)
- The identification of the part of the Code most relevant to the activity
- Evidence that you undertook the CPD activity

Sounds pretty straightforward? …or are you struggling? Let's go back to Michelle and her revalidation.

This is Michelle's continuing professional development log. The key here is to add to this list each time you undertake any training or development programmes to avoid being bombarded when adding everything and trying to remember dates the month before your revalidation is due (or complete the revalidation notebook I suggested).

Dates:	Method Please describe the methods you used for the activity:	Topic(s):	Link to Code:	Number of hours:	Number of participatory hours:
14/06/2020	Intermediate life support training at General Hospital	Emergency life support.	1–19	2 hours	2 hours
20/10/2019	Work shop induction to General Hospital: lecture/workshop (once)	Sepsis, deteriorating patient, documentation, falls safety, under water sealed drains, temporary pacing boxes, pharmacy overview, pain management.	1–25	8 hours	8 hours
10/01/2020	Corporate induction: lecture-based (once only)	Induction to the General Hospital	10, 20–25	3½ hours	1 hour
23/03/2020	Introduction to patient handling- e-learning and practical learning	Safe and effective moving and handling procedures/ correct protocol and use of moving and handling devices.	1–19	8 hours	6 hours
03/04/2020	Fire training: lecture-based	Policies and procedures of fire safety and what to do in the event of a fire at work.	1–19	3 hours	1 hour
03/04/2020	Data protection: lecture-based	Principals of protecting sensitive data and the nurse's role in this.	1–25	4 hours	1 hour
14/03/2020	Administration of intravenous medications: lecture and personal learning with preceptor	The administration of intravenous medications- theory and practical, including a self-assessment	1–19	6 hours	3 hours

Continued

Dates:	Method Please describe the methods you used for the activity:	Topic(s):	Link to Code:	Number of hours:	Number of participatory hours:
04/04/2020	Administration of medications: lecture-based, and on ward discussion with pharmacist	Policies and procedures, and the principles of safe and effective medication administration.	1–25	3 hours	1 hour
04/04/2020	Infection prevention and control: lecture-based	Principals of effective infection prevention and control and the nurse's role.	1–19	3 hours	0 hours
04/04/2020	Medical gases awareness: lecture	Administration of medical gases.	1–19	2 hours	1 hour
04/04/2020	Safeguarding children: lecture	Principals of how to safeguard children	1–25	3 hours	3 hours
04/04/2020	Anaphylaxis: lecture	How to manage anaphylaxis	1–19	3 hours	3 hours
04/04/2020	Patient group directions: lecture	A look into discharge planning and implementation of community support referrals	1–19	2 hours	0 hours
06/04/2020	Right patient, right blood: Theory lecture-based	Theory behind the administration of blood products	1–19	4 hours	2 hours
06/04/2020	Adult safeguarding: lecture	Principals of how to safeguard adults	1–25	3 hours	3 hours
07/04/2020	Tissue viability: lecture	Principals of wound care/ management	1–19	2 hours	0 hours
07/04/2020	Health and safety awareness: lecture	Principals of achieving effective health and safety in the workplace.	1–25	2 hours	1 hour

Dates:	Method Please describe the methods you used for the activity:	Topic(s):	Link to Code:	Number of hours:	Number of participatory hours:
07/04/2020	Legal and professional issues related to record keeping: lecture	Principals of effective record keeping	1–25	3 hours	0 hours
13-17/05/2021	RCN virtual Congress: debates, lectures and active involvement with other registrants (voluntary)	Widening perspective on nursing and nursing-related issues	1–25	40 hours	40 hours
25/09/2021	Heart and lung sounds: lecture	Osculation of chest, heart and lung sounding	1–19	7 hours	3 hours
19/10/2021	Enteral feeding lecture	Safe and effective administration of enteral feeding	1–19	7 hours	3 hours
14/01/2021	Epidural and PCA training: lecture and practical assessment, Genera Hospital Pain team office A-block	Pain management devices	1–19	3 hours	3 hours
11/04/2021	Immediate life support in education centre	Emergency life support.	1–19	6 hours	6 hours
23/04/2021	ALERT Course in education centre	Recognition of deteriorating patient	1–19	7 hours	7 hours
24/05/2021	Fire training update: on ward	Policies and procedures of fire safety and what to do in the event of a fire at work.	1–19	1 hour	1 hour
29/05/2021	Urinalysis training for new devices on ward	Use of a new device for obtaining urinalysis from patients	1–19	30 minutes	30 minutes

Continued

Dates:	Method Please describe the methods you used for the activity:	Topic(s):	Link to Code:	Number of hours:	Number of participatory hours:
21/05/2021	Supervision one, on ward	To assess my ability to carry out my nursing duties	1–19	1 hour	1 hour
18/06/2021	Supervision two, on ward	To assess my ability to carry out my nursing duties	1–19	1 hour	1 hour
18/06/2021	Appraisal, on ward	To assess my ability to carry out my nursing duties	1–19	1 hour	0 hours
18/09/2021	Aseptic non-touch technique, on ward	To assess my abilities in carrying out aseptic non-touch techniques needed for tasks such as wound dressings and administration of intravenous medications.	1–19	1 hour	1 hour
10/04/2021	Hyponatraemia, E-learning	To assist me in understanding how to assess, treat and diagnose a patient suffering from hyponatraemia.	1–19	2hour	1 hour
17/05/2021	Cannulation and venipuncture education centre	How to obtain blood samples and insert intravenous cannulas.	1–19	4 hours	2 hours
15/06/2021	Delirium raining on ward	Lecture on how to nurse the patient suffering from delirium and the trust the policies and protocol in this.	1–19	1 hour	1 hour
				Total: **160.80**	Total: **105.5**

The NMC doesn't outline particular details of CPD activity for you; it allows you to make the decision about what areas you feel will help to enhance and improve your practice. Completing these CPD activities doesn't mean you need to go back to the classroom. On occasion, this may be the case to achieve participatory activities. However, you can also undertake CPD activities online (most of us have become experts in this as a result of the pandemic).

As far as evidence goes, keep all the certificates you get when you complete training or any handouts/printouts which may prove you have actually done what you said you have (remember the saying in nursing, *'If it isn't written, it hasn't been done'*). Put this information in your portfolio for safekeeping (it may also be of use if you want to refresh your knowledge one day). You could also reflect on your training and use this towards your revalidation, but we will discuss this later in this chapter.

Are things starting to make more sense now?

If they aren't, browse the NMC website for step-by-step videos and discussions with practitioners who have undergone the revalidation process. You could also take a look at the NMC guidance sheet: https://www.nmc.org.uk/globalassets/sitedocuments/revalidation/examples-of-cpd-activities-guidance-sheet.pdf

Blank copies of all the templates you need for your revalidation can also be found on the NMC website; http://revalidation.nmc.org.uk/download-resources/forms-and-templates.html

Now, let's tackle step three…

PRACTICE-RELATED FEEDBACK

Over the course of your career you will receive feedback on you as a nurse and your abilities. This feedback may come in the form of a thank-you card from a patient and their family as you discharge them home, or from a discussion with your colleagues about the help you gave them during a difficult experience.

Feedback may also come in the formal circumstance of an appraisal or a letter from management. Whatever the form of feedback, it is all useful in your revalidation and to help you develop in your role as a nurse.

For revalidation purposes, you must obtain five pieces of feedback over the course of three years from when you last renewed your registration or from when you qualified. If you obtain verbal feedback, take a note of what the feedback was, where it happened and who it was from. Put this in your portfolio along with any cards, letters or notes you receive in relation to your practice.

Good feedback is always great to hear. It gives you that ego boost, that good feeling that *'Yeah, I can actually do this.'* It is a useful tool in telling you how you are doing and what others think about you as a nurse.

Just like good feedback, bad feedback also plays an important role. Bad feedback can come out of a situation where, maybe, you didn't handle things well, or you felt overwhelmed, because you needed to refresh your knowledge on a certain topic.

Receiving this type of feedback will make you reflect on your practice and should give you that boost to improve. So if it is something that helps make your practice better, consequently improving patient experiences and outcomes, then why not use it in your revalidation?

Let's take a look at how you should log your feedback for the revalidation process…

NMC feedback log:

Date	Source of feedback Where did this feedback come from?	Type of feedback How was the feedback received?	Content of feedback What was the feedback about and how has it influenced your practice?
23/06/2021	A letter from deputy charge nurse Sam	Charge nurse Sam presented me with a letter outlining a discussion he had with a patient's relative, which highlighted successes in the care I provided.	This letter outlined an occasion where a family member had praised the care that I had provided for their relative, describing me as *'a credit to the profession'*. This feedback was wonderful to hear and has given me confidence in the care I am providing, making me feel valued as a nurse. In addition, by receiving a letter from my manager, I also felt appreciated as a member of the team. This has positively influenced my practice by giving me more confidence and helping me believe in myself more.
15/12/2021	A letter from my ward manager.	My ward manager presented me with a letter outlining a discussion she had with a patient's relative which highlighted successes in the care I provided.	This letter outlined an occasion where a patient had praised the care I had provided for them describing me as *'a credit to the profession'*. This feedback was wonderful to hear and has given me confidence in the care I am providing making me feel valued as a nurse. In addition, by receiving a letter from my ward manager, I also felt appreciated as a member of the team. This has positivity influenced my practice by giving me more confidence and helping me believe in myself more.

Date	Source of feedback Where did this feedback come from?	Type of feedback How was the feedback received?	Content of feedback What was the feedback about and how has it influenced your practice?
Over the past 3 years	A collection of cards from patients and family members.	A collection of thank you cards from patients and family members from the past 3 years.	These cards from my patients and their families are the best feedback I have received, as it tells me that I am doing my job well and that patients and their families are happy and satisfied with the care I have provided. This has positively influenced my practice by giving me more confidence and helping me believe in myself more.

Above are three examples of feedback and how you may want to log them in your portfolio. Remember, you need five pieces, so next time you receive a compliment or have a constructive conversation about your practice with someone, write it down, log it here, and you'll be set by the time your revalidation comes around.

WRITTEN REFLECTIVE ACCOUNTS

After reading Chapter three, you should be a pro at reflecting by now. As we discussed, reflection is a big part of becoming a safe and effective practitioner because it helps you to strengthen your critical thinking skills; the reason you choose to do something and why, which will, in turn, allow you to identify any changes required to improve your others' practice. All of which will help to enhance the care provided and received.

Reflection is also a massive deal when it comes to your revalidation. Just like feedback, you need five reflections, all written by you, based on experiences you've had over the past three years. These reflections can be about anything, from the drug error you made in your first week as a newly registered nurse (we all make them) to the time where you performed cardiopulmonary resuscitation (CPR) for the first time. Like feedback, these reflections can be based on the good, the bad and the ugly (let's face it, nursing can be all at some stage) as long as you're honest and develop strategies in your reflections which will help to learn, improve and perfect your nursing abilities.

The NMC tells us that our five reflections can:

- Be about your CPD, and/or
- A piece of practice-related feedback you have received, and/or
- An event or experience in your own professional practice.

AND…. how they relate to the code, it's simple really (see, this revalidation business isn't as scary as everyone thinks…right?).

The NMC again provides you with reflection templates, which are the forms you fill in, which will help you to write and shape your reflection. You can use these templates or, of course, write in whatever way you feel most comfortable.

Just fill in the little boxes (see example below) to explain to your confirmer what your reflections are about (you don't have to show them the whole reflection if it's something you're not comfortable sharing with that person, but do have them handy on the day you revalidate to prove you have actually completed them).

'By reflecting and linking it to the code, it will make me more aware of the code in my everyday practice and help me to use it in the decisions I am making each day.'

Let's look at how Michelle prepared her reflections for her revalidation using the NMC's templates:

Reflective account:

One: based on practice-related feedback

What was the nature of the CPD activity and/or practice-related feedback and/or event or experience in your practice?

Charge nurse presented me with a letter outlining a discussion they had with a patient's relative, which highlighted successes in care I provided during a particular busy period on the ward.

What did you learn from the CPD activity and/or feedback and/or event or experience in your practice?

I have learnt from this feedback that I am doing a good job and that I need to have more confidence in my abilities, skills and decision-making. This feedback also highlights that my hard work hasn't gone unrecognised and that I am supported by management on the ward.

How did you change or improve your practice as a result?

This letter outlined an occasion where a family member had praised the care I had provided for their relative, describing me as '*a credit to the profession*'. This feedback was wonderful to hear and has given me confidence in the care I am providing, making me feel valued as a nurse. In addition, by receiving a letter from my manager, I also felt appreciated as a member of the team. This has positively influenced my practice by giving me more confidence and helping me believe in myself more. This feedback has changed my practice, as I believe I am more confident and assertive in my role as a staff nurse and now don't always second-guess myself when I have a feeling that a patient is deteriorating and ask for another opinion. I am now able to recognise this without question and act accordingly.

How is this relevant to the Code?

Select one or more themes: Prioritise people – Practise effectively – Preserve safety – Promote professionalism and trust.

This feedback has helped me to work within all aspects of the Code as it reflects my ability to prioritise people as demonstrated in the feedback. The patient's relative explains how I made not only the patient but the entire family feel at ease when their relative began to deteriorate and that I was fast and efficient in acting accordingly when this occurred. I practised effectively in how I implemented care that assisted in helping that patient to improve their condition and did so to a high standard. This is reflected in how the feedback states that I am a '*credit to the profession*'. I preserved patient and family safety by implementing care immediately, which was relevant, necessary and effective. I did all of this while acting in a professional manner, which assisted in my patient and their family trusting me and my abilities as their nurse.

It is important to remember when reflecting that you do not record any information which can be used to identify another person in order to protect their confidentiality.

'I wasn't concerned with the actual reflection, as I know I do this every day; it was writing it down and constructing a written reflection that worried me…I'm not a good writer at the best of times, and getting my feelings and thoughts written in a professional way was overwhelming. I spoke with my colleagues, and together we realised that we don't need to write a book, we just need a few simple lines of what happened and how it had influenced or changed our practice…Using the NMC template really helped me construct what I wanted to say in a formulated and professional manner.'

REFLECTIVE DISCUSSION

This section of the revalidation process involves discussing with another person on the NMC register your five pieces of feedback and your five reflections. This area of the revalidation process has been designed to help practitioners talk about their practice and identify areas where they can improve. Reflection allows you to think about an experience or a situation and how it has affected you. Discussing this with someone else can assist you in developing plans or strategies to improve and deal with similar things again by learning from each other and putting your refection into everyday practice.

The NMC states that the reflection discussion 'is designed to encourage a culture of sharing, reflection and improvement by:
- Requiring you to discuss your professional development and improvement
- Considering the role the standards in the Code have in your practice and professional development
- Ensuring you don't work in professional isolation
- Giving you the opportunity to respond constructively to feedback, experiences and learning'.

The person who you choose to have your reflective discussion with doesn't need to be the same person as your confirmer. This person does need to be on the NMC register as another nurse, midwife or nursing associate. So…if your manager is a nurse on the NMC register, then why not do both your reflective discussion and confirmation with them? Keep it simple.

HEALTH AND CHARACTER

The health and character declaration is simply you making the NMC aware of any criminal convictions or cautions you may have been charged with. If you haven't, you simply state that you're in the clear. If you have, you need to make the NMC aware of this in accordance with the Code.

PROFESSIONAL INDEMNITY ARRANGEMENT

Both the health and character declaration and the professional indemnity arrangement are completed online. They are simple tick-box exercises with space to add details as required. No need for templates, reflections or discussions here.

In terms of professional indemnity, as a registered nurse, you are legally required to have an arrangement in place in order to practices. Usually, your employer will have this arrangement made for you, but it is worth checking to confirm this.

Confirmation

Well guys, you've almost done it! You are on the final step of completing your revalidation! This is the part where you've completed all of the reflections, you've had your discussion, you've logged all your CPD and practice hours and filled in those certificates…now you need to go through everything with your confirmer and get all those important details, i.e. their name, PIN (or relevant professional identification number), their professional address and email. This, for them, is a real 'sign your life away moment,' which is why you need to make sure you've got everything in order!

Your confirmer will declare that you have completed everything that the NMC has required you to do in order to meet the revalidation process. There is a form this person needs to fill out, and you should keep it safe in case the NMC requires it at any stage. Once you and your confirmer have had your face-to-face discussion, and they are satisfied enough to sign everything, you go online and submit your application. Your revalidation discussion needs to be completed in the last year of the three-year period in which your revalidation falls in order to be as recent as possible. You then submit the application at least 60 days before your revalidation date (you'll find this information online on your NMC profile; the NMC may also email you or send out a letter with this information).

And folks….that's it. You've achieved it. You've completed the dreaded revalidation process. It's not as scary or daunting as it seems…right? It's actually a pretty rewarding experience if you prepare in advance and give yourself enough time to enjoy it.

Just remember how fast university went, how fast each placement went….wait and you'll see how fast three years of being a nurse go and you'll be thankful that you kept your portfolio up-to-date.

Nursing Associates

The term, nursing associates, has been around for a few years now. A lot of people still find it hard to understand what it means and who these mysterious people are (especially because they only exist in England at the time of writing). Well…let's investigate them a little so next time you're on shift and your colleague is a nursing associate, you'll understand their role and their scope of practice a little better.

In recent years, nursing associates have been able to register with the NMC for the first time. Their primary role in England is to support nursing and bridge the gap between registered nurses (that's you) and healthcare assistants. Nursing associates are just as accountable to the NMC as you are, but they usually work under your direction (you being the registered nurse).

Nursing associates work in almost all areas of health, from general practice surgeries to community, hospital and mental health. They have been trained via an apprenticeship programme through university and placement (something like your nursing degree, but only over two years and maybe with a little less detail).

Nursing associates can perform many clinical tasks, including obtaining blood samples, insertion of cannulas, electrocardiograms (ECG's), performing and recording clinical observations, supporting patients and their families with bad news, and recognising and reporting adult/child safeguarding issues.

Nursing associates can go on to become nurses, but they will need to undertake a nursing degree via a university. However, due to their prior education and experience, the time frame may be reduced.

Find out more information on nursing associates on the NMC or RCN websites.

Our Moment in History: The COVID-19 Pandemic

People often say you remember where you were the moment something monumental in history happened, like when Neil Armstrong took those iconic first steps on the moon or when the horrifying images of President John F Kennedy, shot in Dallas, Texas, hit our TV screens. More recently, we remember hearing of the death of Queen Elizabeth II or even where we were when we saw the first images of the 9/11 attacks on the United States. These memories, whether we lived through them or not, are etched in our minds forever.

And then came 2020. Who could have ever predicted the seismic events which would impact our world forever. From a few cases in Wuhan, China, to a local outbreak, followed by an epidemic, then a pandemic, the world once again watched in fear. The coronavirus pandemic prompted governments all over the world to act in order to protect their people. Soon came the lockdowns; businesses shut their doors, and we were told to cover our faces and stay apart. In the United Kingdom (UK), the government told its people to *'Stay Home, Protect the NHS, Save Lives'*. It was a mantra designed to stall the virus spread, prevent hospitals from becoming overwhelmed and buy time for preventative or reactive treatments to emerge, or so it was hoped.

The weeks and months passed, cases rose and so too did deaths. Health officials warned of near-apocalyptic scenes. Even after a period when cases fell, the easing of government restrictions on businesses reopening and on social interaction brought with it further waves, more cases and more deaths.

In the UK, the coronavirus pandemic was described as the country's worst crisis since the Second World War. In her address to the nation, the Queen recalled the famous wartime song *'We Will Meet Again'* in an effort to rouse people's spirits, unite their efforts behind the government's restrictions and remind them that better days would return. The emergency also drew comparisons with the Spanish influenza, which struck after the First World War, killing millions as it rapidly spread. This flu is estimated to have killed more people than those who died during the conflict which preceded it. It was therefore feared that coronavirus would do the same.

However, this time, the frontline was not the trench or the battlefield; it was the ward, the intensive care unit (ICU), the nursing home and our own homes.

Instead of the soldier geared in uniform holding weapons, it was the nurse and the doctor draped head-to-toe in visors, gowns and gloves who had to lead the fight, this time against an invisible enemy. Rather than going home to barracks, the frontline fighters returned day after day to their families, often in terror that they were unwittingly bringing the enemy home to those they loved the most.

For what felt like countless hours and endless days, staff sweated through personal protective equipment (PPE) and experienced trauma, loss and scenes they will never forget.

As the pandemic raged, PPE became a growing concern. Would there be enough? Would health care workers be and feel safe going onto wards with the infected patients? Would the global demand cause prices to soar and the frontline suffer?

The rest of the world was told to stay at home, but this was not an option for healthcare workers. Instead, these individuals were sent into the battlefield unsure of the weapons they could use, terrified they would lack protection and, no matter what happened, knowing they would be in the firing line.

At the start, staff faced the unknown. This new virus was different. Treatments and therapies that were once standard practice to deal with a deteriorating patient were simply not enough anymore. Every day a new symptom of the virus emerged, from a cough, to high temperature, to the loss of taste and smell. This was no ordinary virus, or at least one that staff were trained for.

Intensive care workers were the first to be called upon. Their skills were not only invaluable but also in high demand. Anyone with this level of experience was drafted into dedicated coronavirus hospitals and wards. It was a time when COVID-19 was the dominant medical need and other surgeries and treatments would have to wait.

Throughout the past 11 chapters, we have taken a journey together to help prepare you for your new life as a registered nurse. However, there are some things you cannot prepare for. No book, or lecture could fully prepare anyone for what was about to unfold in the year 2020. Instead, what we will do in this chapter is tell you about the real-life, lived experiences of nurses who worked during one of the most monumental moments in the history of the health service.

We will explore the journey of four different nurses, including the author of this book, about their varied experiences working during the pandemic. They will detail the impact it has had on them and reflect on what lessons they hope nurses can learn in the future. The pandemic truly was an event that has the potential to change the healthcare service and nursing as we know it. It may take a long time before this impact can be fully assessed.

One nurse, Niamh Garland, a theatres nurse, was redeployed to a COVID intensive care unit (CICU), where she spent the better part of a year nursing patients with COVID-19. While working in CICU, Niamh describes her experience as *'Really tough, it took its toll on everyone. Some nurses I have worked with for years will never be the same again.'*

Catherine McLaughlin is another nurse who joined the already strained workforce in tackling COVID-19. Catherine was a final-year nursing student when the pandemic first hit and overnight took on her new role, months earlier than she had anticipated. Catherine, who is now a staff nurse working in Vascular Surgery, describes her first few months of working as a newly registered nurse as *'nerve wrecking'* and *'traumatic'*.

Suzanne Tauro, an experienced clinical research nurse, describes her contribution to work during the pandemic as *'worthwhile'* and *'meaningful'*. As a stroke clinical research nurse, Suzanne helped to deliver life-saving treatments to patients attending hospital with a stroke. During the pandemic, Suzanne was tasked with the hefty job of leading a team in contributing to research into the treatment and preventative measures in tackling this new disease.

Joleen McKee, the author of this book and also a registered nurse, was redeployed during the pandemic to help deliver care in the private sector. As COVID numbers increased, life-saving surgeries were reduced and in some instances ceased. In order for patients to receive their *'last attempt at treatment'*, the private sector now opened its doors to National Health Service (NHS) patients.

As the cases rose, staff from all areas were moved where the need was greatest. The call went out to retired and former medical professionals in the hope they could use their experience to backfill shifts. It was all hands on deck. Even students were given a baptism of fire. With health wards no longer the place for guided learning, many stepped up to the mark and had to fill the shoes of a registered nurse overnight.

In the early days, governments planned for extra facilities to house patients, such was the anticipated number. Grimly, plans were also in place for mass morgues. Our modern times were thrown into a crisis of biblical proportions.

In the UK, the images from northern Italy, of hospitals overwhelmed and deaths spiralling out of control, made people heed the advice. But this was not an issue consigned to one country or region. The virus reached every part of the world, and quickly.

Niamh Garland was one such nurse who had to answer the call when the pandemic began:

In the initial stages of the pandemic, there was so much confusion and fear of the unknown. Firstly I was told I was needed to go work in one hospital, then suddenly it changed to another. There were lots of management meetings, but staff on the ground really didn't know what was going on.

Before March 2020, Niamh was a highly trained and skilled theatres nurse working at Belfast City Hospital (BCH). But that was all about to change. Because of her abilities, Niamh, along with her colleagues, was always going to be among the first to be called upon when this unforeseen medical crisis emerged.

Some of the tasks would be similar, but this was facing into the unknown, with patients' lives in your hands and, when the long shifts ended, on your mind too.

Because of the nature of this disease, families were not allowed to be with their loved ones during their last few moments. It was the nurses who were there, strangers or not; it broke my heart every time I saw a patient die knowing their loved ones were so close yet also so far away.

In theatres, Niamh was used to intense pressure and extremely sick patients. Some, because of the nature of their surgeries and conditions, could emerge worse from operations. Sometimes as a nurse, your best efforts can only do so much. Coronavirus, for many nurses and doctors on the frontline, would see such cases increase greatly. For the best efforts, these were sick patients, and there was little that could be done to help them.

Let's take a look at Niamh's story to get a better idea of what she really experienced.

Redeployment and Moving to the Frontline

Before becoming a nurse, Niamh worked as a care assistant in a nursing home. Niamh completed her nursing degree in 2016 and, following a successful management placement in theatres at the BCH, took up her first role as a registered nurse there. In the years leading up to the pandemic, Niamh worked with patients undergoing various surgeries but did not have any real ward-based experience since registering. As such, she was notably worried about her role in nursing patients with coronavirus.

Niamh says she and her colleagues were '*scared about COVID*'. This extended from the experienced staff to those who were still learning their trade, across every discipline. As she describes, from '*nurses to doctors and anaesthetist*', it was a new experience and one they were struggling to get to grips with. '*This disease was so new, and we didn't really know anything about it, so it was hard to prepare yourself for looking after these patients.*'

By the time the first patients were admitted to Niamh's hospital with COVID-19, staff knew they would not be like any they had cared for before. Niamh describes that despite her training and experience, she and her colleagues did not feel ready for this new challenge: '*As much as our skills and knowledge were to a high level, we were not ICU nurses and doctors, we were not intensivists.*'

In the run-up to working in the BCH Nightingale (re-purposed Covid hospital), Niamh explained that she and her colleagues felt tense, on edge and worried about what lay ahead of them. They were petrified they were going to contract this deadly disease or, worse, infect those they loved.

Niamh describes that she and her colleagues even bought wellie boots: '*We were so scared that we bought wellie boots so we could tuck our scrubs into them so that we were covered all over in PPE. We didn't want any chance of the disease going onto our socks or our ankles. Some staff even used hairspray to ensure every strand of hair was tucked away. We were told COVID could sit on your hair and your skin, and if you unknowingly touched it then you could spread the disease.*'

Niamh explains that she '*showered at work after taking off PPE*'. Staff were advised to do this as a means to protect themselves and those they would come into contact with outside work. While PPE is highly effective in managing exposure to the virus on a ward, it can only do so much.

'*When I got home, I stripped off at my back door, had another shower straight away and made sure to wash everything properly*', she continued.

'*I didn't want to spread this infection, so I took all precautions I could.*'

Niamh describes her training in preparation for taking on her new role. *'We only had a few hours of training with an ICU nurse who talked us through a head-to-toe exam of a patient.'*

Niamh states she was told during this training and when in discussions with management that she and her theatres nurse colleagues would only be *'support nurses to the ICU nurse; we would carry out clinical duties we were trained for to help ease the ICU nurses' workload'*. However, this isn't how things worked out.

> *The support nurse idea wasn't a reality. My first shift in ICU was a nightshift, and I was left to deal with a patient on my own.*

It was known that during the height of the pandemic, staffing levels were over-stretched, and on some occasions staff were forced to work under immense pressure and carry out tasks they weren't familiar with.

Despite Niamh's array of skills and training, intravenous (*IV*) drug administration was not something she required for her role as a theatres nurse:

> *I don't have ward experience, I didn't even have intravenous drug administration training, and yet I was left to deal with syringe pumps and ventilators I had never even seen before.*

Niamh says that she was *'scared'* of COVID-19 *'like everyone'*.

However, she adds, her *'real fear'* was feeling underprepared. She says the patients who needed treatment for the virus were *'so sick and on so many different drugs that I wasn't familiar with'*.

> *I had never used some of the machines they were on and I was terrified I was going to do something wrong which would harm my patient. I lived shift by shift and minute by minute with constant fear and anxiety.*

However, Niamh's experience was not unique. Social media blew up with accounts from doctors, nurses and allied health professionals telling their stories of feeling overwhelmed and underprepared for this new virus. Many explained that they had either not received enough adequate training to help assist them in the roles they were redeployed into or that there was simply not enough of them to deal with the increasing demand of patients requiring intensive care treatment.

Every nurse understands the pressures that the healthcare service comes under every winter as flu season takes hold, or people suffer injuries during colder weather, but 2020 was on another level. This time, the pressure did not subside, and only intensified as winter turned to spring and spring turned to summer, with the system facing sustained pressure like never before.

For nurses, the pressure manifested itself in many ways. Niamh says she felt *'vulnerable and at risk'* not only of contracting this deadly disease but also of prosecution if her actions to save patients' lives were not enough.

We were told that during the pandemic we would have to adapt our skills, other-wise our patients would suffer.

Niamh further explains that this sometimes meant she would have to learn new skills, and quickly so that her patients' care was not compromised: *'I had to do it to keep my patients alive.'*

Like Niamh, so many others faced these same challenges where they needed to step up in order to protect their patients and assist in helping the healthcare service to survive this unthinkable crisis.

Catherine McLaughlin is another nurse who, like Niamh, worked during the pandemic under immense pressure. However, unlike Niamh, Catherine was a final-year nursing student when the pandemic first hit and joined the frontline in a baptism by fire.

I was eager to help, but I was terrified as I didn't know what I was up against.

Let's dive into Catherine's experience of becoming a nurse during a pandemic.

A Baptism by Fire: The Student Experience

In the UK, as coronavirus cases rose, so too did the admissions to hospital. Clinics, wards and office spaces were converted into ICU bedspaces to house patients struggling with this disease. The call went out to anyone with medical training to help if they could. Students were among those asked to step up and join the frontline.

Catherine McLaughlin had to go from student to staff nurse overnight. After considering nursing as a career from a young age, she eventually decided to apply to join the profession following a positive interaction with her health visitor after the birth of her sixth child. As a mature student and mother, Catherine says she is *'robust and used to dealing with life's challenges'*; however, she never anticipated that her career would take such a turn so quickly, never mind before she had even registered.

Catherine, who decided to join the frontline when the call went out to students, states she was *'eager to help'*, yet she felt *'frightened about what lay ahead of her'*. As a confident student, Catherine felt she had the skills and knowledge to make a contribution; however, like many students, she was concerned that her skills were still at a raw stage to be utilised on the frontline without support from a preceptor.

As we discussed in Chapter four, the preceptorship process gives you the opportunity to get familiar with your new area of work, your colleagues, the routine and everything that goes into being a successful and effective nurse. However, Catherine's experience was different. The already overstretched and underfunded healthcare service now faced new challenges associated with the devastating effects of COVID-19. Staff were redeployed, leaving some areas short on the ground. What this meant for Catherine was that she didn't always have the luxury of an experienced nurse to help guide her through her first few weeks and months. Instead, Catherine was expected to fill the gap.

Looking back now, Catherine describes her experiences as *'traumatic and frightening'*. Although she does praise her ward and the staff who she worked with, she acknowledges that during the pandemic there was less support made available to her as a result of the staffing problems and added pressures that COVID-19 placed on the healthcare service.

Like all healthcare workers who served during the pandemic, Catherine was worried about bringing the virus home, particularly as two of her children were in *'high risk'* categories. One has diabetes, while the other has asthma.

The mother-of-six says her husband's attitude was *'we just have to be careful'*, but this is easier said than done when dealing with a medical threat evolving day by day. *'It was a hard decision to work on the wards at this time'*, she explains.

> *We only went food shopping, but we were good at staying in, there were risks everywhere.*

Catherine says she would change clothes at the back of the house after arriving home from work, dividing her house into sections so she could safely avoid her family until she could wash and get changed.

> *It was always at the forefront of my mind and contributed to stress.*

She adds that she has *'never done so much reflection in my life'* due to the circumstances she faced.

Despite all the precautions, one of the worst-case scenarios became reality: Catherine tested positive for COVID-19. Through all the precautions, the PPE and keeping her distance, the virus still managed to infect a student nurse trying her best to avoid it. Catherine's case happened during the first wave of coronavirus in 2020.

'Two nights I woke up and felt like a bus was parked on top of me', she details.

However, unlike many who required hospitalisation, Catherine's symptoms were *'luckily mild'*.

Some of the student nurse's family were also tested, with negative results. Somehow, isolated in her bedroom, she did not infect her family.

'My priority was my children', she says. *'I felt like I failed them by bringing this home.'*

It was not Catherine's fault that she tested positive, but she says she *'constantly berated'* herself after receiving the result.

'We were so thorough with our PPE on the ward', she continues.

Like many other areas in the health service, Catherine worried about the supply of PPE. *'There were times we were close to the wire'*, she continues, *'I had to be fit-tested multiple times as the masks were changing and some were running out of stock.'*

The stress and added pressure of the supply of PPE to help protect Catherine so she could in turn protect her patients and her family caused anxiety and worries, leading to incidents where Catherine *'cried in the staff bathroom'*.

As we discussed in previous chapters, the period of being a newly registered nurse is intense and stress-filled, with the added worries and pressures associated with the

COVID-19 pandemic; it was not surprising Catherine experienced a decline in her mental health. This decline saw Catherine seek refuge with her line manager, who supported her and told her to *'stop being so hard on yourself'*.

Other colleagues reassured Catherine that she was performing well and she should not expect to have the same level of know-how as those who had several years of nursing experience.

She says she had an element of *'imposter syndrome'*, not believing she belonged as a nurse at such a time.

Catherine, who is *'very competitive by nature'*, wanted to do better and be the best nurse she could be. So discussions and support from her manager and her team were *'invaluable'*, she says.

Teamwork in nursing is key. Suzanne Tauro, a clinical research nurse, knows all too well how important good teamwork and effective communication can be, especially when leading a team while conducting a clinical trial for a vaccine which would *'help us and our families return to some sort of normality'*.

Let's take a look at what Suzanne experienced during the pandemic.

Treatments and Vaccines: Could We End the Lockdowns?

Suzanne is a nurse who has vast experience. Despite working on trials which have contributed towards life-changing and life-saving treatments, she says she was *'nervous she didn't have the skillset'* to enter the battle against a pandemic, but was *'willing to do what she could'*.

Suzanne explains that during the early phases of the pandemic *'everything was up in the air'*. Following multiple meetings with management, clinical trials were suspended in all areas apart from the concerted focus on finding ways to tackle COVID-19.

As the medical world sought strategies to get to grips with the virus, it became clear that vaccines offered some hope of stemming its spread and providing the world with a route out of lockdowns. Suzanne was one of the nurses tasked with conducting trials with patients who were willing to participate in vaccine studies. Without them, history could have been very different. Vaccinations for COVID-19 have undoubtedly prevented many deaths and given hope at a time when all seemed lost.

'I felt like I was doing something really worthwhile,' she comments.

Suzanne further states that she was *'emotional'* when family and friends told her they were *'proud'* of her contribution to the research.

Previously part-time and with two young children, Suzanne made the decision to increase her hours in work, so determined was she to play her part.

Furthermore, the Tauro family's efforts in the COVID-19 fight continued with Suzanne's husband, a doctor who worked on wards helping coronavirus patients.

Despite her valuable role in the fight against coronavirus, Suzanne says she felt *'ashamed and embarrassed'* that her duties were not by the bedsides of patients. At a time when the health service was '*on its knees*', managers declined calls by Suzanne to let her work on the frontline, even though she would have been '*nervous*' to do so. On reflection, Suzanne realised her managers were thinking of the bigger picture.

She states: '*They needed us to be available to work on trials to help deliver treatments on vaccines which would free us from the pandemic.*'

To allow Suzanne and her husband to carry out their work, Suzanne's parents took on childcare responsibilities. For parents across the health service, childcare, during a period when schools and nurseries closed, became an added worry.

While Suzanne was grateful that her parents could step in, she says she had the constant worry that through this interaction she was placing them at risk.

'*It is scary, we are all only human*', Suzanne explains.

This was the first time in my career I wished I wasn't a nurse because I was really scared to go to work.

The author of this book, also with clinical research experience, shared Suzanne's worries about attending the hospital environment at work and what that could mean if she became infected and went on to spread the virus to others.

Working on a clinical trial which hoped to identify different drugs and treatments in the care of ICU patients with COVID-19, the author felt proud to contribute towards developments in battling this new virus. However, despite seeing results first hand, caution remained, and the worry that the trials may not lead to an end to the nightmare of the pandemic.

All over the world, scientists and researchers directed their focus to the pursuit of developing treatments for COVID-19. Even though some methods proved successful, it took many months for due process, through trials and studies, for the world to hear the news that certain treatments, drugs and therapies would begin to show improvements in the care of patients with COVID-19.

However, despite the advancements beginning to show light at the end of the tunnel, many patients who did not contract this deadly disease also suffered devastating losses due to the pandemic. As COVID-19 took hold, governments began to reduce output services in the healthcare system, which meant a knock-on effect for those living with terminal and life-altering conditions. As a result, some private healthcare services now offered their support.

The author of this book was one of many nurses redeployed onto the frontline in the private sector during the pandemic.

Public to Private Sector: The Author's Experience

When COVID-19 first began to show its presence in the NHS, I was working as a staff nurse in a cardiothoracic Surgery pre-assessment unit. Here, patients were pre-assessed and supported through all stages in preparation for their open heart and thoracic surgeries.

We first heard of the novel coronavirus and thought it felt like miles away in China. However, the more and more the cases there were, and the more the virus spread, we realised we may need to move to the frontline in order to help assist in the delivery of care for our patients.

As my background is cardiothoracic surgery, I was first sent back to the ward where I had worked for years. This time things felt very different. Surgeries were beginning to be cancelled, the amount of PPE we required began to increase, and soon we saw our first few cases of COVID-positive patients come through our doors. My anxiety levels began to increase. I was confident in my abilities to work on this ward, to nurse critically ill patients following major surgery. However, I feared the unknown. I worried that we would not have the capacity to care for these new patients coming in with COVID, but I was also concerned about what would happen to our already sick and vulnerable patients sitting on waiting lists for life-saving surgeries.

I worked a few shifts on the ward before being redeployed to the private sector to help train and support staff who would now be nursing *our surgical patients*. One hospital in particular opened its doors to our surgeons and our patients during the pandemic, so some of those awaiting their life-saving lung cancer surgery could be given their chance at treatment.

During the initial stages in the private sector, I felt grateful that our patients were getting the treatment they needed; however, I was concerned that we still had many thousands awaiting the same call for surgery.

As the days and months passed, I began to realise just how infectious COVID was. My father, awaiting a transplant at the time, and my mother, who lives with cardiac issues as well as diabetes, were always at the forefront of my mind. As the restrictions became tighter, my worries heightened. How would my parents access food supplies and their own medical treatments and support? Could I potentially carry COVID to them through my food deliveries and socially distanced medicine drop-offs? Would I be able to forgive myself if anything happened to them because I worked on the frontline and could not stay home to look after them? After all, I have the skills and knowledge to do so.

As a relatively new nurse myself, I still have the fire inside me to be the best nurse I can be and to always put the patient first. However, during a pandemic we must not forget that while the patient is priority, you the nurse must remember you are just as important. You must realise that if you are not protected, not only in adequate PPE but also from stress and burnout, then you cannot be the saviour the press promotes you to be, the 'angel' saving lives and putting the needs of others above your own.

During the COVID-19 pandemic, many of us witnessed trauma, loss and scenes of devastation. We worked under immense pressure never before experienced by our health service. It is therefore not surprising that many medical professionals experienced declines in mental health; many changed forever.

Will anyone ever be the same after COVID?

Let's take a look at how COVID-19 has impacted our mental health and changed us as a society forever.

Who Cares for the Carer? Mental Health Challenges, COVID-19

During a career in nursing, everyone will experience incredible highs and unbearable lows. There is elation and satisfaction when you know your work contributes towards a patient getting better. However, there are other times, and not necessarily a reflection on your skills, when a patient may get more sick, or die, while in your care. It can make you doubt your confidence and talents, and even make you question if you are cut out for the role. It is in every moment, in good times and bad, that looking after your mental health and well-being is of paramount importance.

COVID-19 stretched health professionals to the limits, both in their abilities to work and their abilities to cope. This book was written with COVID-19 fresh in the mind. It could be years before some healthcare workers, believing they dealt with its stresses well, come to realise that they too need support because of the trauma they endured.

Niamh Garland says she got through the experience *'hour–by–hour'* and felt *'no support'*.

'We sat constantly in fear', she says. Niamh watched as a colleague left work for months, suffering from post-traumatic stress disorder (PTSD) – a condition which many people who work in healthcare will face, and one which was amplified by the pandemic.

> *Nurses have been changed, and many do not have confidence in their own abilities anymore. It was luck of the draw if you have had a semi-OK experience or whether it has changed you forever. My colleague hasn't been the same since.*

Each person will find their own ways to deal with stress and difficulties. There is no prescribed easy method to handle challenges to our mental health. Niamh says she often *'bottled up'* the *'emotional turmoil'* she was going through.

However, at a time when the pandemic was the primary concern, she says her focus was on *'doing all you can to look after those patients'*.

> *I would come home and be an emotional wreck and be crying, thinking of the patients who died, not having a dignified death.*

> *I felt like I had let my patients down.*

Niamh's advice for newly registered nurses, or those entering such a crisis in the future is: *'Remember you need to care for yourself too.'*

> *It's very easy to paint on a smile even if you're not OK. You don't know what's going on in other people's lives. Put yourself in their shoes and be there for your colleagues too.*

She adds: *'Nursing is challenging at the best of times, never mind COVID; take time to look after your own mental health so you can keep going.'*

Catherine McLaughlin says nurses need more support and that she has had many days *'so bad'* she feels unable to talk about it when she comes home to her family.

Complaining that the health service is under-funded, under-staffed and under-resourced, she says further backing by government would *'improve those days'*.

It gets embarrassing hearing the term, hero, about nursing.

It also amplifies our position and makes us vulnerable. If we make a mistake, it's terrible, as it's not something that can be lived up to.

Catherine says she would *'think a lot'* about the clap for carers and tributes to healthcare staff which were lauded during the pandemic, particularly in the first wave of COVID-19.

She says while she appreciates the sincerity of the support which was offered, healthcare staff *'are human too'*, and this can be taken away when viewed as *'heroes and angels'*.

It was a challenging time, she explains, getting to grips with the job during a crisis, but like most times when you deal with sick patients, *'it is worth everything'* when they reach out and tell you that *'you're an asset to nursing'* because you cared for them.

Learning Lessons

The point of this chapter is to make you, the reader, think and acknowledge that the future is unpredictable and that only by learning lessons and assessing the experiences of those who came before can we be prepared for similar things that could happen in the future.

The NHS and the wider world were not prepared for COVID-19, despite some models and experts fearing that such a virus could take hold, and with all the major incident and emergency procedures and planning we were still not ready. There is no way to know if a similar virus or one that spreads faster or is more deadly could emerge again in the future.

None of the nurses we heard from in this chapter trained for the pandemic. They entered nursing with the simple goal of making patients better; it just so happened that COVID emerged on their watch and they did the best they could.

Yes, healthcare workers are heroes, but not the invincible types from Marvel or DC comic books. Rather, they are emotional heroes, skilled and prepared to do the best they can. They are also vulnerable heroes.

To be the best nurse, you need to realise you will not always have the answer, and in times when the work environment gets too much, or when other issues in your life affect your work, asking for help is not a weakness. It is a strength, and one which will only make you stronger.

Handing Over

Whether you are a student about to enter the world of nursing, someone who has started their first tense days seeking reassurance or with experience and seeking a refresher, I hope this book has offered some comfort and encouragement.

I want the main takeaway to be: You are not alone.

Every nurse has been there. We all started somewhere, sometime, with the same fears and anxieties, many of which never truly subside.

Perhaps you are overwhelmed with worry, questioning, *'Am I good enough? Can I really do this?'*

I have asked myself these questions multiple times, and I know I am not alone in that.

The answer I want you to remember: You are good enough and you can do it.

Throughout this book we have discussed how to master the interview, and how preceptorship can help to make that transition from student to nurse.

We have examined how you can ease into this demanding world and what to do when things go wrong.

Nursing is constantly evolving, and all of this will change as time goes on, but at the core, the focus of what we do is helping others.

When times are tough – and they will feel unbearably tough on occasion – remember why you wanted to be a nurse, remember why you started.

Nursing is undoubtedly the lifeblood of healthcare, perhaps even the nation.

With our skills and devotion, nurses care for the sick and provide crucial interventions to keep people well.

Our service never ends.

It is rarely advised to think about work in your downtime, but take a moment now and again to consider nurses in far-off places who at any given time are saving lives and providing comfort.

From state-of-the-art complexes in major cities to makeshift tents in tiny villages, each nurse has a duty to uphold the integrity of this most noble profession and serve the patients who need us.

But – and it's a big but – we do this job often stressed and strained to our every sinew, and quite often starved of resources.

Giving up would be the easy option – but we continue because we care.

Many health workers have felt encouraged by the 'clap for carers' and the heightened respect for the NHS which emerged during the COVID-19 pandemic.

It was a moment many will cherish – but make no mistake, this can subside. We have to fight as nurses to be heard, sometimes calling out bad practice, sometimes telling those in authority that we need more to do our job effectively.

We fight for the patient. We fight because one day we, or those dearest around us, could be the patient.

There is no quick fix, but as new nurses, this is, sadly, the reality.

Here is the job advert you will not read:

Welcome to a lifestyle that will bring you tears; some happy and some sad. There will be laughs and fun, smiles and joy along the way, but they will dovetail with moments of sorrow and frustration, while being pushed to the limitats of what a human being can witness or deal with.

There will be countless memories too, some good, others you wish you could let go of.

But – there is no other job like it.

It is hoped this book has provided an encouragement, not a deterrence.

This is truly a remarkable job, and it should be a badge of honour.

One theme I hope that has hit home is that, with each experience, there is further experience to gain. It is a mantra which, if kept in mind, can keep your feet on the ground. No matter how good a nurse you are or will become, remain humble.

The world of medicine and healthcare has evolved beyond recognition in recent decades. We do not know it all; no one ever will.

There will always be new discoveries, new training and fresh ways to improve our care to help patients get better quicker and be supported when they leave our sight. That is why reflection is considered so important and features so prominently in this book.

Keep notes, remember the difficult decisions you made and why. Always question if you can improve, or, with hindsight, what you would have done differently.

Above all, please take away from this publication a recognition that nursing is a team game. We are only as good as the people we call upon for support; they are our colleagues, our friends and help. Our band of brothers and sisters.

It should always be about the patient – if we all pull together, this job with long hours will not feel like work, but a vocation you were born to do.

To conclude, this is something I wrote during one of my first days; it is something I trust will sound familiar to many readers.

It's 06:00 and my alarm rings, disturbing a restless sleep where I was already half awake to watch the sun rise and hear the first chirps of birds in the trees outside.

I threaten to turn over, too exhausted.

06:03 – the first of my three-minute interval alarms shrieks at me to 'Wake up!'

Ok, ok, and I wake, resenting the thought of lifting my head from the pillow.

It's 06:15 now and the dread begins. I'm getting ready, but am I really ready for this, all over again?

It's 06:45 and I'm riddled with anxiety. Some excitement to see people again – I wonder who's on shift and what the day will bring – but also, the anxiety. The worry.

I feel bluer than the blue tunic I pull on, crisp and fresh from my mother's ironing. I felt bad texting her last night to ask if she didn't mind as once again I was 'sorry, I'll not get away on time'.

It's 06:50, my palms are wet and my mouth feels dry. Was there a point in ironing this? I can already feel like I'm sweating. What if I make a mistake? What if today is a disaster?

It's 07:00, I force myself out the door, knowing in half an hour I need to accept the keys to my medicines trolley. It will be stocked with drugs ranging from simple pain relief and anti-sickness medications to the finest antihypertensives that keep blood pressure at a satisfactory rate.

What if the man in bay four is even sicker? What if the woman in side room two is going to yell at me again?

It's 07:15, minutes before I look at the tired, sad and fragile faces, while being told about their conditions and what kind of night they had. It's not even eleven hours since I left them.

It's 07:25, I walk through the door. It flaps behind like I'm entering a wild west saloon.

I'm in, I'm the nurse.

I look around and see the tunics, many like my own. There are the doctors, the support staff, the managers, the kitchen staff taking breakfast orders.

It's nearly time for the hand-over.

Goodness knows what the day will bring, but I'm a nurse now, I can do this. And I wouldn't have it any other way.

Thank you for taking the time to read this book, and I wish you the best of luck in your journey as a nurse. You got this!

Now, let's really begin.

BBC. (2021). *West Suffolk Hospital hunt for whistleblower 'incendiary' says report.* Retrieved from https://www.bbc.co.uk/news/uk-england-suffolk-59597801.amp

Centres for Disease Control and Prevention. (2021). *The U.S. Public Health Service Syphillis Study at Tuskegee.* Retrieved from https://www.cdc.gov/tuskegee/timeline.htm

Data Protection Act. (2018). Retrieved from https://www.legislation.gov.uk/ukpga/2018/12/contents/enacted

Equality Act. (2010). Retrieved from https://www.legislation.gov.uk/ukpga/2010/15/contents

Gibbs G. *Learning by doing: A guide to teaching and learning methods.* Oxford Oxford Polytechnic; 1988.

Health and Safety at Work Act. (1974). Retrieved from https://www.legislation.gov.uk/ukpga/1974/37/contents

Johns C. *Transforming nursing through reflective practice*, 2nd ed. Wiley-Blackwell; 2005.

Mental Capacity Act. (2005). Retrieved from https://www.legislation.gov.uk/ukpga/2005/9/contents

National Health Service. (2022a). *NHS Jobs.* Retrieved from https://www.jobs.nhs.uk.

National Health Service. (2022b). nhsjobs.com. Retrieved from https://www.nhsjobs.com

National Health Service, Stress. (2019). Retrieved from https://www.nhs.uk/mental-health/feelings-symptoms-behaviours/feelings-and-symptoms/stress/

Nightingale F. *Notes on nursing: What it is, and what it is not.* New York: D. Appleton and Company; 1860.

Nursing and Midwifery Council. (2018). *Realising professionalism: Standards for education and training.* Part 2: Standards for student supervision and assessment. Retrieved from https://www.nmc.org.uk/globalassets/sitedocuments/standards-of-proficiency/standards-for-student-supervision-and-assessment/student-supervision-assessment.pdf.

Nursing and Midwifery Council. (2019a). *Part 1: Standards framework for nursing and midwifery education.* Retrieved from https://www.nmc.org.uk/standards-for-education-and-training/standards-framework-for-nursing-and-midwifery-education/

Nursing and Midwifery Council. (2019b). *Guidance sheet - Examples of CPD activities.* Retrieved from https://www.nmc.org.uk/globalassets/sitedocuments/revalidation/examples-of-cpd-activities-guidance-sheet.pdf.

Nursing and Midwifery Council. (2019c). *Revalidation/resources: Forms and templates.* Retrieved from http://revalidation.nmc.org.uk/download-resources/forms-and-templates.html.

Nursing and Midwifery Council. (2020a). *Standards for nursing associates.* Retrieved from https://www.nmc.org.uk/standards/standards-for-nursing-associates/

Nursing and Midwifery Council. (2020b). *Principles for preceptorship.* Retrieved from https://www.nmc.org.uk/globalassets/sitedocuments/nmc-publications/nmc-principles-for-preceptorship-a5.pdf

Nursing and Midwifery Council. (2022). *What is revalidation?* Retrieved from https://www.nmc.org.uk/revalidation/overview/what-is-revalidation/

Nursing and Midwifery Council, Reflective Discussion. (2021). Retrieved from https://www.nmc.org.uk/revalidation/requirements/reflective-discussion/

Protection from Harassment Act. (1977). Retrieved from https://www.legislation.gov.uk/ukpga/1997/40/contents

Public Interest Disclosure Act. (1988). Retrieved from https://www.legislation.gov.uk/ukpga/1998/23/contents

Rolfe G, Freshwater D, Jasper M. *Critical reflection in nursing and the helping professions: A user's guide*. Basingstoke Palgrave Macmillan; 2001.

Royal College of Nursing. (2019). *NMC: Preceptorship*. Retrieved from https://www.rcn.org.uk/get-help/rcn-advice/nursing-and-midwifery-council-precept.

Royal College of Nursing. (2020). *Revalidation*. Retrieved from https://www.rcn.org.uk/professional-development/revalidation.

The Disability Discrimination Act. (1995). Retrieved from https://www.legislation.gov.uk/ukpga/1995/50/contents

The Nursing and Midwifery Council. (2018). *The code*. Professional standards of practice and behaviour for nurses, midwives and nursing associates. Retrieved from https://www.nmc.org.uk/globalassets/sitedocuments/nmc-publications/nmc-code.pdf

Wong-Baker FACES Pain Rating Scale. (2001). Retrieved from https://www.ghc.nhs.uk/wp-content/uploads/CHST-Wong-Baker-Pain-Scale.pdf

Note: Page numbers followed by *t* and *b* indicate tables and boxes, respectively.